Robert E. Our famili...
Amy Ad... ...*Squire S...*
Editors

Our Families, Our Values
Snapshots of Queer Kinship

Pre-publication
REVIEWS,
COMMENTARIES,
EVALUATIONS . . .

"***O****ur Families, Our Values* is a strong, multifaceted response to the bigotry and ignorance that today fuels the virulent and all too often violent 'culture wars.' But at the core of many of its chapters is the celebration of real partnership—and thus real family values—community, empowerment, pleasure, and love."

Riane Eisler
Author, *The Chalice and the Blade, Sacred Pleasure,* and *The Partnership Way*

"***O****ur Families, Our Values* provides an amazing array of 'snapshots of queer kinship.' It is to be praised for its breadth of vision, bringing together authors from so many different religious worlds and so many different queer perspectives.

These essays will make you think about what families and values really are; about the ways those terms are brought together in our society to have only one meaning; and about why we need to think in more daring and expansive ways about families and values."

Rabbi Rebecca T. Alpert, PhD
Co-Director, Women's Studies Program,
Temple University,
Philadelphia, PA

More pre-publication
REVIEWS, COMMENTARIES, EVALUATIONS . . .

"The chorus of voices of queer kinship cries out for not only recognition of the particular patterns of gay, lesbian, bisexual, and transgendered lives, but a thoroughgoing redefinition of terms of relationship. Friendship, marriage, family, tradition, desire— all are broken open, expanded, and reformed around the wide repertoire of queer personal and community experiences. New terminology springs up where the old fails: *blendship, mother-in-love, co-parent, at-home-ment.*

The angel of religious scripture is wrestled with and compelled to yield a blessing to supercede the wound it has long inflicted. Rather than defend the hackneyed passages from Jewish and Christian Bibles that are used to admonish the gender-transgressive, the authors search out positive texts for trailblazing, gender-adventurous lives.

If there is a unitive theme in this collection that ranges from cheerleading and affirmation to challenge and prophetic heralding, it is courage. We hear of the gay couple for whom HIV is the third companion of the relationship, and of a Jewish rabbi and congregation attacked for encouraging 'anti-Jewish lifestyles, sin, and abomination' that creates a ritual rainwater bath for a man with AIDS forbidden entry to the local *mikvah*. We hear of households daring to parent children that society might snatch from them. We are challenged to ruminate whether even the bar and bathhouse sex of the urban gay community might serve unitive, community-forming, traditional functions that invite scrutiny and moral evaluation by religious communities that have, in the past, dismissed them unexamined. We are called, again and again, to think, to talk, to consider what fresh fusion of old and new ideas, values, morals, and practices can be life-giving."

Rev. Dr. Jennifer M. Phillips
Rector, Trinity Episcopal Church,
St. Louis, MO

"A compassionate, dynamic presentation of the lifestyles of gay, lesbian, bisexual, and transgendered people. It is read through tears, laughter, pain, and acceptance of all lifestyles. Through the experiences of the writers, there is deep appreciation for the sexual preferences of all people."

Rev. Evlyn W. Fulton
Retired clergy,
Presbyterian Church,
St. Louis, MO

The Harrington Park Press
An Imprint of The Haworth Press, Inc.

Our Families, Our Values
Snapshots of Queer Kinship

HAWORTH Gay & Lesbian Studies
John P. De Cecco, PhD
Editor in Chief

Our Families, Our Values
Snapshots of Queer Kinship

Robert E. Goss
Amy Adams Squire Strongheart
Editors

The Harrington Park Press
An Imprint of The Haworth Press, Inc.
New York • London

Our families, our values

Published by

The Harrington Park Press, an imprint of The Haworth Press, Inc., 10 Alice Street, Binghamton, NY 13904-1580

Cover design by Monica L. Seifert.

Library of Congress Cataloging-in-Publication Data

Our families, our values : snapshots of queer kinship / Robert E. Goss, Amy Adams Squire Strongheart, editors.
    p.   cm.
    Includes bibliographical references and index.
    ISBN 1-56023-910-7 (alk. paper).
    1. Gay male couples—United States.   2. Lesbian couples—United States.   3. Gay men—United States—Family relationships. 4. Lesbians—United States—Family relationships. I. Goss, Robert. II. Strongheart, Amy Adams Squire.
HQ76.3.U5093 1997
306.84'8—DC21
                                       97-1311
                                          CIP

To all who shared themselves in this book,
their families, and friends.

*   *   *

In memory of Edward Gray Squire, Jr.

*   *   *

To Laura Elizabeth Bryte Squire

CONTENTS

ABOUT THE EDITORS

The Reverend Robert E. Goss, ThD, is a faculty member of the Department of Religion at Webster University in St. Louis, Missouri. An activist and former Catholic priest, he is the author of *Jesus ACTED UP: A Gay and Lesbian Manifesto* (HarperSanFrancisco, 1993). He is a co-founder of Food Outreach, St. Louis, a food service organization that provides meals and nutritional supplements to persons living with HIV. He has been active with ACT UP in both St. Louis and Boston and works with the Treatment Issues Group of ACT UP. In addition, he has transferred his clergy credentials to the Universal Fellowship of Metropolitan Community Church, where he is clergy on staff in St. Louis and is involved in the training of future MCC clergy. Dr. Goss is Co-Chair of the Gay Men's Issues in Religion Group of the American Academy of Religion. He received his doctorate in theology and comparative religion from Harvard University.

Amy Adams Squire Strongheart is a gay civil rights activist, public speaker, writer, and editor. Her commentaries, book reviews, interviews, and news stories have appeared in over a dozen publications, including the *St. Louis Post-Dispatch*, for which she writes a regular guest commentary on lesbian and gay issues. She is a member of the National Lesbian and Gay Journalists Association and is a board member of Other Sheep: Multicultural Ministries with Sexual Minorities, an international ecumenical ministry to lesbians and gays. In 1991, when Ms. Strongheart and her life-partner were joined in the first public same-sex union in the Episcopal Diocese of Missouri, she legally added the chosen name "Strongheart."

CONTRIBUTORS

Rev. Dr. Mary L. Foulke is the Protestant chaplain at Wellesley College in Wellesley, Massachusetts. She completed her doctorate in religion and education at Union Theological Seminary in New York City and Teachers College/Columbia University in New York.

Rev. Dr. Thomas Hanks, currently living in Latin America, is an Old Testament theologian from Concordia Seminary (St. Louis, Missouri). He has taught in Costa Rica and Argentina. A Presbyterian, Hanks is author of *God So Loved the Third World* (Maryknoll: Orbis Books, 1983) and Old Testament editor of the *New Illustrated Dictionary of the Bible* in Spanish (San Jose/Miami; Caribe, 1968). Dr. Hanks is currently executive director of Other Sheep (*Ministerios Multiculturales con Minorias Sexuales*). He is the father of two children.

Dr. Richard P. Hardy, is a professor of spirituality in the Faculty of Theology, Saint Paul University, Ottawa, Ontario, Canada. Dr. Hardy has taught and lectured in Canada, the United States, Asia, and Europe. He has taught graduate courses on AIDS and spirituality in Ottawa as well as at the Graduate Theological Union in Berkeley, California. Besides workshops and conferences on spirituality and persons living with HIV/AIDS, he has also published several books and numerous articles on spirituality, including *Knowing the God of Compassion: Spirituality and Persons Living with AIDS* (Ottawa, ON: Novalis, 1993).

Rev. Dr. Renee L. Hill is an assistant professor of theology and director of studies in feminist liberation theologies at the Episcopal Divinity School at Cambridge, Massachusetts. Hill is the author of "Who Are We for Each Other: Sexism, Sexuality, and Womanist Theology" in *Black Theology: A Documentary History, Volume II 1980–1992,* James H. Cone and Gayraud S. Wilmore (Eds.) (Maryknoll: Orbis Books, 1993). She completed her doctorate in systematic theology at Union Theological Seminary in New York City.

Dr. Mary E. Hunt is a feminist theologian who is co-founder and co-director of the Woman's Alliance for Theology, Ethics, and Ritual (WATER) in Silver Spring, Maryland. She is a Roman Catholic in the women-church tradition who lectures and writes on theology and ethics with particular attention to liberation issues. Hunt is the author of *Fierce Tenderness: A Feminist Theology of Friendship* (Crossroad, 1990), which was awarded the Crossroad Women's Studies Prize for 1990. She is the editor of *From Woman-Pain to Woman-Vision: Writings in Feminist Theology by Anne McGrew Bennett.* Among her many publications are chapters in several books, as well as articles in the *Journal of Feminist Studies in Religion, America, Concilium, Conscience, The Witness, Open Hands*, and *Second Opinion.*

Michael Bernard Kelly was born in Melbourne, Australia, and studied theology and spirituality at Melbourne College of Divinity and at Holy Name College (Oakland, California). He is the author of *The Erotic Contemplative: The Spiritual Journey of the Gay/Lesbian Christian*, a video course published by Erospirit Research Institute in 1994. He was recently interviewed for *The Fall Upward: Spirituality in the Lives of Lesbian Women* (Little Gem Publications, 1996), a new book examining the lives of twenty Australians working in gay spirituality. Mr. Kelly has extensive experience as a retreat leader, ritualist, and spiritual director in both Australia and the United States, and has also trained and taught with Joseph Kramer in erotic spirituality. He seeks to live as an openly gay, contemplative man, and on the margins of the Catholic community. He divides his time between the United States and Australia, where he lives in a small coastal town outside Melbourne.

Victoria S. Kolakowski is a lesbian transsexual patent attorney, political and religious activist, and minister-in-training. She holds two master's degrees in engineering (electrical and biomedical), a master's degree in public administration, and a law degree, as well as a certificate in theological studies from the Pacific School of Religion in Berkeley, California, where she is pursuing a master's degree in divinity and a master of arts degree. Kolakowski is a candidate for ordination in the Universal Fellowship of Metropolitan Community Churches and is student clergy at New Life Metropolitan Community Church in Berkeley. She co-authored Berkeley, California's domestic partner registration system for the general public.

Joseph Kramer is founder of The Body Electric and head of Eros/ Spirit Research Institute. Kramer has a master's degree in divinity from Jesuit Berkeley School of Theology. HBO did a thirteen-part series called *Real Sex*, and Joseph Kramer was the topic of one of those segments.

Rev. Leng Leroy Lim is from Singapore. He is the Episcopal chaplain at the University of California at Los Angeles, curate at St. Bede's at Marvista, and a health outreach worker with the Asian Pacific AIDS Intervention Team in Los Angeles. He received his master of divinity degree from Harvard University Divinity School. He wrote "Exploring Embodiment" in *Boundary Wars: Intimacy and Distance in Healing Relationships*, edited by Kathrine Ragsdale (The Pilgrim Press, 1996). Leng is interviewed in Doug Sadowick's *Sex Between Men: An Intimate History of Sex Between Men, Postwar to Present* (HarperCollins, 1996). Lim's dream is to organize a queer group on an expedition to the Arctic.

Eric Rofes teaches and is a doctoral student in social and cultural studies at UC Berkeley's Graduate School of Education. He founded the Boston Lesbian and Gay Political Alliance, and served as executive director of the Los Angeles Gay and Lesbian Community Services Center and San Francisco's Shanti Project. He is the author of seven books, most recently *Reviving the Tribe: Regenerating Gay Men's Sexuality and Culture in the Ongoing Epidemic* (The Haworth Press, 1995).

Dr. Kathy Rudy is assistant professor of ethics and women's studies at Duke University. She is the author of *Understanding the Ethics of Abortion: Moral Views in Competing Communities* (Beacon Press, 1996) and *Sex and the Church: Gender, Homosexuality, and Contemporary Christian Politics* (Beacon Press, 1997). She is interested in ethical issues pertaining to both Christianity and feminism, and is especially concerned with problems related to gender, homosexuality, and medicine.

Singing Cow (Sonia-Ivette Roman) is a Wiccan high priestess and leader of Polyhymnia, a Gardnerian teaching coven in New York City. She is also an elder of The Covenant of the Goddess, an international organization of Wiccan covens. In addition to her extensive training in the mystical arts, she is also well-versed in pastoral counseling techniques. She has taught workshops on world mythology, Wicca, and African diaspora religions. Her articles have appeared in *Harvest, Our Pagan Times,* and *Frighten the Horses.* She was also the contributing editor of the mythology, religion, and music sections of the latest edition of the *Barron's Concise Student Encyclopedia.* She is a proud Puerto Rican.

Rev. Dr. Jane "Janie" Adams Spahr earned both master of divinity and doctor of ministry degrees from San Francisco Theological Seminary in San Anselmo, California. She is currently lesbian evangelist for "That All May Freely Serve," a mission project of the Downtown United Presbyterian Church in Rochester, New York, in partnership with Westminster Presbyterian Church in Tiburon, California. Spahr is one of four editors of *Called Out: Voices and Gifts of Lesbian, Gay, Bisexual, and Transgendered Presbyterians.* She is the mother of two, a teacher, learner, preacher, and friend.

Dr. Elizabeth Stuart is senior lecturer in theology at the University of Glamorgan in Wales. She is the author of a number of works on lesbian and gay sexuality and theology, including *Daring to Speak Love's Name: A Lesbian and Gay Prayer Book* (Hamish Hamilton/ Viking, 1992); *Chosen: Gay Catholic Priests Tell Their Stories* (Geoffrey Chapman, 1993); *Just Good Friends: Towards a Lesbian and Gay Theology of Relationships* (Mowbray, 1995); and *Christian Perspectives on Sexuality and Gender,* with Adrian Thatcher (Fowler Wright, 1995). She is executive editor of the journal *Theology and Sexuality.* She is a Roman Catholic and member of the Universal Fellowship of Metropolitan Community Churches.

Dr. Michael J. Sweet is a psychotherapist at the Mental Health Clinic of the Madison, Wisconsin VA Hospital and a clinical assistant professor in the Department of Psychiatry, University of Wisconsin-Madison. He received PhDs in Buddhist studies and counseling psychology, both from the University of Wisconsin-Madison, and is a licensed psychologist and clinical social worker. He has published articles on psychotherapy, Buddhist meditation, and the history of sexuality. Sweet is currently working with collaborators on two books: one on queer identities in classical Indian culture, and a translation and study of two Tibetan mental purification (*blo sbyong*) texts.

Rabbi Susan Talve is the rabbi of Central Reform Congregation in St. Louis, Missouri, and a co-founder of and spiritual resource for the St. Louis Gay and Lesbian Chavurah. She has long been a heterosexual ally to the lesbian, gay, bisexual, and transgendered community. She is also a wife and mother.

Rev. Dr. Mona West received her PhD in Old Testament studies from Southern Baptist Theological Seminary in 1987. She taught biblical studies at Austin College in Sherman, Texas, and at Anderson College in Anderson, South Carolina. Currently, West is the academic dean of the Samaritan Institute for Religious Studies, which is the professional school of the Universal Fellowship of Metropolitan Community Churches. West's most recent publications include "Ruth," "Song of Songs," and "Lamentations" in the *Mercer Commentary on the Bible* (Mercer Press, 1995).

Rev. Nancy L. Wilson is the author of *Our Tribe: Queer Folks, God, Jesus, and the Bible* (HarperSanFrancisco, 1995) and *Amazing Grace*, with Malcolm Boyd (Cross Press, 1991). Wilson is senior pastor at the Metropolitan Community Church of Los Angeles and vice moderator of the Universal Fellowship of Metropolitan Community Churches. She has previously served as the ecumenical officer to the Fellowship. Wilson was first elected to the Universal Fellowship of Metropolitan Community Churches Board of Elders in 1976 and has subsequently been reelected to four consecutive terms. Wilson lives with her spouse of eighteen years, Dr. Paula Schoenwether, in the Los Angeles area.

Rev. Brad Wishon, formerly pastor of Metropolitan Community Church in St. Louis, has had the privilege of working with dozens of lesbian and gay couples as they prepared to formally celebrate their relationships. He has acted as pastoral advisor on issues pertinent to healthy relationships, has helped to find solutions to problems couples are experiencing, and has sought to provide input to the community on building healthy relationships through the experience he has garnered. He has been a guest speaker at Eden Seminary in St. Louis, on the topic of pastoral counseling for gay and lesbian couples and has advised mainstream clergy on how to serve their lesbian and gay members who seek to have their relationships publicly blessed. Wishon is currently the pastor of Gentle Shepherd Metropolitan Community Church and is working on his PhD. He lives with his partner Mark.

Preface

In this last decade before the dawn of a new millennium, those of us who are of the Lavender Tribe* have come to understand the term "family values" as the code phrase for legislation and social policy that would outlaw our families and drive us all underground. Many have been led astray by the notion that to promote and protect Lavender relationships and kin is to somehow detract from the legitimacy or importance of the so-called traditional family,** which actually accounts for an astoundingly small percentage of family groupings globally.

In the late spring of 1996, our state representatives introduced HB 1637 into the Missouri legislature. It reads in part: *The child welfare policy of this state is what is in the best interests of the child. There is a rebuttable presumption that homosexual, bisexual, transsexual, and transvestite parents are unfit to be awarded custody of children under 18 years of age. In order to rebut this presumption, a homosexual, bisexual, transsexual, or transvestite parent must prove fitness for custody by a preponderance of the evidence.* This sadly misguided and mean-spirited bit of drivel was blithely marketed to Missouri citizens under the guise of "family values."

This is hardly an isolated case. In anticipation of a ruling from Hawaii recognizing the legitimacy of same-sex unions, legislators across the nation are falling over each other in their haste to pass bills to make such unions illegal in their various jurisdictions. In September 1996, Congress overwhelmingly passed the Defense of

---

* Transgendered, transsexual, bisexual, lesbian, gay, a person with AIDS, or one who loves any of us.

** A traditional family consists of a married woman and man who are presumably heterosexual, although heterosexuality is not a requisite if their gayness is well-closeted. The couple has between one and four happy, perfect, drug-free children who are neither adopted nor related through a previous marriage. The woman stays at home to rear the children, and the man is the "breadwinner" and the "head of the household."

Marriage Act (DOMA), which defined gender requirements of spouses. DOMA will go down in history as one of the low points in our nation's struggle with social bigotry.

Even William Jefferson Clinton and Hillary Rodham Clinton, by far the most compassionate, progressive, and Lavender-friendly couple ever to occupy the White House, have failed to advocate strongly for the rights of Lavender people, despite many campaign promises to do so. In the dead of night, without cameras or microphones to record his shame, President Clinton signed DOMA into law.

Our congressional representatives thumbed their noses not only at gay marriage but also at prohibiting discrimination against lesbians and gays in the workplace. The Employment Non-Discrimination Act (ENDA) failed to pass by one heartbreaking vote. In addition, we have witnessed a ubiquitous effort to exclude Lavender people from constitutional protection—Colorado being the most notable of these outrageous efforts, where lesbians and gay men have been murdered outright. We are seeing our rights to life, liberty, and the pursuit of happiness either consistently denied or stripped away one by one.

In the face of these grim tidings, it seems that our fate and the future of our families is in our own hands. It is up to us to recognize and honor the relationships that we hold dear and that we recognize as sacred and familial: that is what *Our Families, Our Values* is about. Grouped into three sections, the essays in this anthology present our imperative to self-advocate by means of the following challenges:

- The first section of essays challenges the widely accepted and seldom contested assumption that only heterosexual people are entitled to get married, have or enjoy sex, or rear children.
- The second group challenges popular interpretations of various scriptures used to perpetuate and justify anti-Lavender injustice and bigotry under the auspices of organized religion.
- The third section challenges the Lavender community, itself, to think clearly and carefully about the course we wish to pursue. For example, how do we wish to define ourselves? Are we really a "people" at all? In what ways do we discriminate against each other? Is it prudent for us to mimic heterosexual

marriage or to define ourselves as "family" when these institutions currently are crumbling under the weight of their own inherent oppressions.

Additionally, as the title implies, this book is an affirmation of those ways in which we do identify as family and of those values that we cherish, such as loyalty, honesty, integrity, humility, inclusivity, service, compassion, and responsibility.

As editors, we have endeavored to put our finger on the pulse of the Lavender Tribe. This volume comprises the viewpoints of twelve women and eight men representing the spectrum of sexual orientations, including lesbian, gay, bisexual, transsexual, and heterosexual. The contributors hail from many hemispheres, and the nations represented are Singapore, the United Kingdom, Canada, Australia, Argentina, and the United States. In addition, these contributors bring a variety of social, ethnic, and religious viewpoints. The faith perspectives reflected in this collection include Wiccan, Jewish, Buddhist, and Christian, both Protestant and Roman Catholic.

Despite the variety of perspectives, you will notice some overlap in ideas, which indicates that for all our differences, we are, in many ways, of one mind. You will also find the usual dissent among the ranks. To be of one mind does not necessarily mean that we must see everything the same way or that we necessarily need the same things.

One thing we do seem to have in common, however, is a sense of grief and outrage over our marginal place in the world. When reading as editors, we take note of what we call the "victim voice," which wails, "Look what those horrible 'others' have done to me." We tried to rein that in or dispense with it altogether because we wanted this book to provide us with some self-awareness and courage to forge ahead. We did not intend for it to give us an excuse to cease taking stock of ourselves, to stop being responsible for our actions, or for failing to do our part to make the world in which we find ourselves a better place. However, we chose to retain much of the sense of personal and collective woundedness. We will never emerge as a liberated people until we have first honored the centuries of pain endured by Lavender folk, and we cannot honor it unless we stop repressing it.

The following pages offer the reader an incredible opportunity to know us in our joy over the welcoming of a child, the blessing of a union, or the finding of oneself, as well as to know us in our sorrow over the loss of a love, the death of a friend, or the betrayal of a culture. These are our families; these are our values.

Robert Goss
Amy Adams Squire Strongheart

Acknowledgments

We thank Cathy Heidemann for her invaluable assistance with manuscript preparation and C. Alexah Strongheart for her indispensable contributions to the development and marketing of this book.

SECTION I.
CHALLENGING PROCREATIVE
PRIVILEGE

Crucial to Lavender liberation is the deconstruction of the following sacred-cow ideologies: that patriarchal families are preeminent over other familial configurations, and that only persons with an opposite-sex orientation and a socially recognized gender identity are entitled to marry, have and enjoy sex, or rear children.

Chapter 1

Queering Procreative Privilege
Coming Out as Families

Robert E. Goss

Procreativity is now used as a weapon by Christian churches to argue theologically against the acceptance of same-sex relationships and, by extension, against the formation of queer families. The procreative bias of Christianity and its imprint on Western culture dissociates queers from family by defining us as outside of procreativity.

When Dan Quayle campaigned for family values, he denounced Murphy Brown as a single mother. When Newt Gingrich preaches about the need for family, he fails to speak of his lesbian half sister Candace. When Jesse Helms thinks of movies reflecting traditional family values, he does not immediately remember *The Adventures of Priscilla, Queen of the Desert*. Throughout American history, the family has been an object of obsessive religious concern. *Family* is a popular term for refuge from chaotic social order, decency, and moral values. Such factors as a high divorce rate, contraception, and abortion have contributed to changes in the social structure of the American family.

The current debate pits the traditional family values of the Christian political right against what it labels as "antifamily" forces. Underlying the debate on traditional family values is the fallacious assumption that queers and families are mutually exclusive groups, set apart without any overlap. Many churches either render our families invisible or abominable. In a wider cultural context, the Christian right has made a programmatic attack on working women; reproductive rights; and the families of ethnic and racial minorities, queers, and the poor, under the slogan of "traditional family val-

3

ues." Their arguments promote an antisexual mentality, obscured by the rhetoric of "family values."

The Christian right suspects that we are subverting the nuclear family, which is the building block for a theocratic society. Most churches claim that the family cannot survive the open social presence of gays, lesbians, bisexuals, and transsexuals. In the late 1970s, gay historian Dennis Altman wrote the following about the homosexual threat: "The homosexual represents the most clear-cut rejection of the nuclear family that exists, and hence is persecuted because of the need to maintain the hegemony of that concept."[1] Our attempts to resignify the family engenders an incredible threat because we defy the customary assumptions about what constitutes family, that is, *Queer* customary notions of family. As Michel Foucault observed, "It is the prospect that gays (and lesbians, bisexuals, and transgendered people) will create unforeseen kinds of relationship that many people cannot tolerate."[2]

Heterosexual liberals and radicals attempted to find alternatives to the nuclear family in the 1960s and 1970s with communes; unmarried couples living together; and diverse forms of political and extended families of choice, crossing ethnic and racial lines. Liberals and radicals recognized that alternative family arrangements were differentiated by culture, class, ethnicity, and lifestyle. Certain liberal groups, such as the Friends of Families in the early 1980s, made a proposal for a "Family Bill of Rights" affirming the right of everyone to create a family form that fits her or his own needs and the right of people to define themselves as families.[3] This bill affirmed the right of gays and lesbians to create families.

The notion of family has been hotly contested within Queer communities. Since Stonewall, there have been many gays and lesbians who accepted the judgment of the Christian right that they represented antifamily forces. Many Queers did not want to duplicate their families of origin, who perhaps rejected them for coming out or who were dysfunctional, operating with unequal gender relations. Some radical lesbians in the 1970s saw motherhood as an oppressive heterosexual institution. The issue appears to have been resolved, as evidenced by the lesbian baby boom of the 1980s and 1990s. Child-rearing has become more common for gay men as they have sought joint custody of their children and developed various strategies for rearing children.

Disagreements still occur over whether or not the Queer movement toward family and marriage rights represents a co-opting into heterosexual society. Are we mainstreaming ourselves into society by adopting the marriage model and by creating families? Some proponents argue that we need the equal right to choose to marry the person we love just as heterosexual citizens can choose. Such a right, they claim, would find greater acceptance of gays and lesbians within society.* Even if the choice were available, some Queers would not marry. I interpret the movement toward Queer marriage rights and family rights as an attempt to mainstream American society to different views of marriage and diverse families.

When I moved in with my lover and life-partner Frank in 1978, we both rejected the model of heterosexual marriage. Marriage was too patriarchal an institution, based on archaic, economic, and oppressive notions of sexual property. We felt that marriage was too dysfunctional a model, patterned after rigid heterosexual stereotypes and unequal power relationships. We did not feel we owned each other, and we did not exchange or hyphenate our surnames. Our heterosexual friends would frequently attempt to gender stereotype us. They would inquire, "Who is the wife? Who is the husband?" There was no wife or husband! We entered into our covenanted love relationship as equal partners, sharing all domestic duties, financial responsibilities, and decision making. We shifted domestic roles, depending on the needs of the moment. Any model for our union had to allow for relational equality, partnership, mutuality, and inclusiveness.

If our relationship was to succeed, we had to create new models for understanding a same-sex relationship and not simply duplicate the heterosexist model of marriage. At that time, there were few visible long-term relationships on which to pattern our own sexual

---

*Andrew Sullivan is the latest voice for marriage rights. He believes that social acceptance of gays and lesbians into the military and their right to marry will allow a virtual equality within society. Sullivan uses the fairness argument for the rights of all Americans to marry, and he maintains that same-sex marriage would foster social cohesion, emotional security, and economic prudence. Andrew Sullivan. *Virtually Normal*. New York: Alfred A. Knopf, 1995, pp.178–187.

love and friendship. Since we both came from the Society of Jesus, a Catholic religious order, we adapted the best aspects of the Jesuit model of friendship, service, and community to comprehend our sexual relationship. We described our sacramental partnership and friendship as a "community of two."[4] Other gay former Catholic clergy have frequently modeled their relationships on the cooperative aspects of teamwork, the sharing of economic resources, and a vision of service embedded within Catholic religious communities.

Our community also exemplified what I characterize as *procreativity,* or rather *Queer procreativity.* We worked with other same-sex couples to develop an interpersonal skills-building weekend, similar to the Catholic model of the marriage encounter. As a Catholic priest, I often blessed many of the unions of same-sex couples who attended this weekend. Yet I was loath, and still am, to call our unions "marriage" because of the gendered property arrangements traditionally associated with marriage. Our unions are frequently more equal than opposite-sex marriages.

Gay, lesbian, bisexual, and transgendered people are openly relating, raising children, and demanding official recognition of their partners as spouses. The current push for domestic partnerships and marital rights in Hawaii challenges the narrow definition of family as two biological parents who are legally married with children.* Interestingly enough, when the reality of the traditional family is critically examined, we find that less than 20 percent of the U.S. population falls into the category of two opposite-sex married parents with 2.5 children.

Narrow definitions, whether from the Christian political right or from Queers themselves, marginalize a number of families in

---

*In May 1993, the Hawaii Supreme Court ruled that the state's refusal to issue civil marriage licenses to same-sex couples under the Hawaii marriage law violates the state constitutional guarantee of equal protection. *Baehr v. Levin,* 852 P2d 44, 74 (Haw 1993). The Lambda Legal Defense and Education Fund has adopted a marriage resolution: "Because marriage is a fundamental right under our Constitution, and because the Constitution guarantees equal protection of the law, Resolved, the State should permit gay and lesbian couples to marry and share fully and equally in the rights and responsibilities of marriage." *The Lambda Update,* 12(1), Winter 1995: p. 7. The Lambda Legal Defense team has initiated the Right to Marry movement within the other states.

America: singles, single parents, divorced and remarried persons, extended families, ethnic families, and all other families of choice. The emergence of same-sex unions in the late 1970s and early 1980s pushed Queer couples in the direction of family roles and the creation of families. For gay men, AIDS may have accelerated the emergence of pair-bonded relationships. The Right to Marry Movement has begun the work of mainstreaming the idea of equal marriage rights, and it has broader social implications for foster-parent adoptions, custody and visitation, and second-parent adoptions.

What I and other contributors to this anthology have to say challenges the last stronghold of Christian patriarchal culture—that of *procreative privilege*. Procreative privilege underpins the Christian cultural notion of marriage and family. Christian church leaders cite procreation as the basis for heterosexual marriage and the family. Historically, Christianity has set married people apart from and against unmarried people. It privileged nonprocreative celibates and elites over procreative married Christians. It also restricted the notion of procreation to opposite-sex marriage only and linked marriage to patriarchal property arrangements. Women remained the sexual property of their husbands. Residual notions of sexual property are ritualized in the marriage ceremony when the father transfers ownership of his daughter to the groom. The bride takes the surname of her husband to indicate that she belongs to him.

Procreativity is now used as a weapon by Christian churches to argue theologically against the acceptance of same-sex relationships and, by extension, against the formation of queer families. The procreative bias of Christianity and its imprint on Western culture dissociates queers from family by defining us as outside of procreativity. For example, in *Bowers v. Hardwick,* Justice Byron R. White concludes, "No connection between family, marriage, or procreation on the one hand and homosexual activity on the other has been demonstrated."[5] For the Christian right and the U.S. legal system, procreativity organizes and structures kinship as a biological family. On the other hand, a New York State of Appeals judge ruled in 1989 that a family can be defined as "two adult lifetime partners whose relationship is characterized by an emotional and financial commitment and interdependence."[6]

While rejecting the nuclear family as normative for all, Queer folks undermine the idea of family as a biological kinship unit, as well as the notion of procreativity. Queering procreativity is a deconstructive process for expanding and redefining family in ways that maintain our rights to difference, equality, family, and sexual partnership. Queering families, moreover, have biblical precedents in the Hebrew and Christian Scriptures.

The Hebrew Scriptures indicate a range of patriarchal families and the construction of some alternative families and diverse households. Family was important to the ancient Hebrews because membership in the Chosen People was authorized through lineal descent. Families were based on patriarchal definitions of women as sexual property and children as human property.[7] There is nothing that approximates a nuclear family within the Christian and Hebrew Scriptures. The only continuity that the contemporary nuclear family shares with biblical families is the patriarchal notion of sexual and human property. The nuclear family, as promoted by the Christian right, represents a capitalist mode of sexual property and human property.

The Gospels dismiss or devalue the family with a number of antifamily sayings, instead prioritizing the establishment of new, alternative families within God's reign.[*] Families in God's reign are reconfigured family, a nonbiological household of equal disciples. Jesus Queered the Jewish household to create families of choice: "Who are my mother and my brothers? Whoever does the will of God is my brother and sister and mother"(Mark 3:31-35). Thus, Jesus redefined the family of God outside kinship lines. The new sisters, brothers, and mothers are without gender hierarchies, status, or economic or political privilege. Jesus seems less concerned with biological families than with the new familial relationships within God's reign. Not even the burial of one's own father was important enough to delay the commitment to discipleship (Luke 9:59-62). Patriarchal fathers are left behind in God's reign (Mark 19:29-30) because God is the only father, voiding the hierarchical position of

---

*Some antifamily sayings are Matthew 8:22, 10:37; Luke 9:60, 14:26. See also Diane Jacobs-Malina. *Beyond Patriarchy: The Images of Family in Jesus*. Mahwah, NJ: Paulist Press, 1993.

all fathers. For Jesus, God does not act like a patriarch. His image of fatherhood is redefined in his story of the prodigal son, in which the father is markedly unpatriarchal in his unconditional acceptance of his son (Luke 15:11-32). Jesus replaced biological families with nonbiological families of faith choice.

Mark (Chapter 10) forms a unified theological excursus on the family, sexual property, issues of power, and hierarchy. Jesus challenged the patriarchal understanding of marriage by claiming that a woman could be turned out from her husband's house by divorce (Mark 10:2-9). *Jesus removed women from the category of male sexual property by his prohibition of divorce and his redefinition of adultery* (Mark 10:10-12). For him, marriage establishes a familial relationship between two persons who are equals in terms of sexual ownership of one another. Jesus also welcomes children into God's reign, removing them from the bottom of the patriarchal family hierarchy and making them persons with their own rights (Mark 10:13-16). When a rich man seeks eternal life, Jesus requires that he give away his property and separate from his family (Mark 10:21).

Even the more distant follower who retains spouse and family must give up the rights of ownership and domination over them. The family is stripped of its unquestioned centrality in the culture and lives of its members, while the adult males who follow Jesus are deprived of status they had enjoyed as heads of such families— all this done "for my sake and the sake of the gospel" (Mark 10:29).[8]

There were two principle institutions in first-century CE Palestine—the family and the state. The patriarchal state depended on the hierarchy of the patriarchal family. Jesus' assault on the patriarchal family, with its sexual property and power arrangements was an assault on the patriarchal state with its notion of property and power. His call of men and women to a discipleship of equals challenged the property and power arrangements of the biological family and, in turn, the Palestinian state under Roman control. Justice, compassion, and love signify the creative presence of God's reign, and any notion of covenanted sexual love between partners needs to include the elements that signify the presence of God's reign. Feminist theologian Dorothee Soelle relates human sexuality to God's reign in the following way: "The greatest project I can name is the quest for justice, what Jesus called 'building the kingdom of God.' Hunger for justice is part of the love energy that is set free in sexual relations."[9] *Genuine sexual love opens the hearts and minds of lovers to other people in need, and this is what Jesus meant by "God's reign."* It is what I call "procreativity."

As previously mentioned, early Christianity set married people against unmarried people. Paul began this separation in his expectation of Christ's imminent return and developed his notions of marriage within that context (1 Corinthians 7:25-40). He begrudgingly allows marriage because it may be necessary to prevent fornication. For the spiritually strong and for Paul, himself, celibacy remained the higher path of holiness. Later, Hellenistic Christians read this Pauline passage from the lens of neoplatonism and Stoicism, and used the concepts to justify privileging the celibate over the married. Celibate monastics would carry on the communal discipleship of equals but would eventually be co-opted into the imperial, hierarchical Church. Marriage would continue to embed property relations. Meanwhile, Paul accepted the notion of human property— slavery and sexual property—as a datum of his patriarchal worldview. He did not fully understand the revolution that Jesus initiated in undermining patriarchal notions of sexual property, children as property, and gender hierarchies. Sexual property has become the contemporary basis of traditional family values, and Christian marriage has been too long a sexual property right for men and male church leaders.

Christianity developed as a religion in the second century CE, at a time when Stoic philosophy, Neoplatonism, and a variety of Gnostic religious movements were primary religious currents in the Roman Empire. Stoicism and Neoplatonism stressed the mind's control over the body, while some Gnostics taught that marriage was either evil or useless. Other Gnostics devalued marriage because the procreation of children was by its nature binding a soul to a body and because matter was considered evil. Gnostic groups generally held one of two extreme positions: either they opposed all sexual intercourse and advocated celibacy, or they advocated all forms of sexual intercourse that were not procreative.

Christian elites sided against sexual intercourse and espoused celibacy. Most Christian writers felt far more comfortable with the ascetic extremist position privileging celibacy as the higher vocation and allowed for sexuality within marriage for the sole purpose of procreation. For Augustine, sexual desire was linked to original sin; thus, marriage became a remedy for concupiscence, or lust, accompanying sin. It was also indispensable to God's plan of salvation for guaranteeing the propagation of humanity. Human sexuality was consequently identified with Stoic norms of procreation and thoroughly disassociated with pleasure. Augustine's position on marriage and human sexuality imprinted both later Catholic and Protestant Christianity's doctrine of procreationism.

Procreationism is a Christian reduction of the purpose of human sexuality to reproduction. It disdains all forms of sexual expression except for penile-vaginal intercourse that is open to conception. Procreationism has become the doctrine of traditional family values. It refuses to understand any variant of sexuality outside of marriage. One evangelical theologian, Thomas Schmidt, writes, "We cannot understand homosexuality, then, simply as a variant of sexuality along the lines of childlessness or celibacy. It is an expression of sexuality contrary to heterosexuality, involving opposing views of the interdependent values of reproduction, complementarity, and responsibility."[10] For Schmidt and many other Christians, Queer sexuality proclaims an independence from the procreative model and thus threatens the traditional Christian definition of family. It is considered to be thoroughly unprocreative and therefore sinful.

Personal fulfillment is often used as a charge against Queers for not engaging in procreativity, or violating or becoming independent of the procreative designs of God. This charge results from a narrow understanding of procreationism, which restricts procreativity to biologicalism and the literal reproduction of human life. Human sexuality is far more than the biological connection of bodies. Procreationism is not procreativity, for procreativity includes, but is not limited to, human reproduction. Several theologians and ethicists assert that gay, lesbian, and bisexual unions can be procreative, that they are not hostile to the regenerative capacities of women, and that they deserve the social recognition of family afforded heterosexual couples by the churches.[11] Procreativity expresses a solidarity with the biblical God who is author of sexual fecundity and justice-love.

Procreativity may refer to the literal renewal of the earth through human reproduction or reproductive strategies, or it may also refer to the contributions made for renewal and transformation of society. Both opposite-sex and same-sex couples have an equal opportunity to express literally and metaphorically the procreativity of the Creator God.

Whom then do we call family? The appropriation of the term *family* is not an assimilationist strategy of finding respectability in general society. *We are not degaying or delesbianing ourselves by describing ourselves as family.* In fact, we are Queering the notion of family and creating families reflective of our life choices. Our expanded pluralist uses of family are politically destructive of the ethic of traditional family values. Critics often charge that our use of family fails to distinguish between biological families and intentional groups or the general community. Their criticism is based on biological definitions of families. Families appeal to many Queers because we came from families. Sometimes, the loss of families of origin through coming out places pressure on some Queer people to recreate families for themselves.

For many, coming out is coming home, belonging to a kinship community or family. Earlier uses of "culture," "subculture," or "ghetto" were impersonal and have been replaced with the personal kinship term of "community." The Queer community has appropriated the notion of community as family for itself when we sing Sister Sledge's song "We Are Family" at our pride festivals. More recently, the notion of community as a family has been replaced with the notion of "tribe" to describe our extended kinship relationship as Queer people.[12]

Contemporary Queers freely choose and create their kinship relationships. Alternative cultural terms for belonging lack the emotional intensity of the term "family," and Queers have been creating kinship groups, households, and families for some time. We use a range of terms to describe the erotic and nonerotic relations that we include in the term family: lovers, friends, parents, fictive uncles and aunts, fictive sisters and brothers, community groups, tribe, and Lavender people. The term family is definitionally extended to couples and singles with and without children, and erotic groups or nonerotic extended families of all types. These are kinship groups of our choice and creation, ranging from erotic coupled to nontraditional erotic relationships and nonerotic relationships.*

Anthropologist Kath Weston speaks of families that Queers "struggle to create, struggle to choose, struggle to legitimate, and . . . struggle to keep."[13] Our new families may or may not live within a household. The complexities of our families of choice are represented by intentional and cultural variables. Families and households often vary in composition, organization, and representation from heterosexual families and households. They vary according to gender, age, class, ethnicity, and sexual orientation. Families consist of household relationships and relationships extended beyond the household: lovers, children, friends. They can include the choice of biological relatives as well. What characterizes these relationships for the most part is that they are chosen.

Deciding who will be part of one's family is a highly personal endeavor. In opposition to the defined notions of a biological family, choice offers the opportunity to recreate and invent the family as pluralistic phenomena without the tyranny of normativity and compulsory heterosexuality. Our choices of families involve all forms of erotic and nonerotic relationships. Since families are chosen, or intentional, we can invent familial forms without the power dynamics, hierarchical assumptions, rigid gender stereotypes, and roles customary to traditional heteropatriarchal biological families.

Those deliberate commitments of Queer singles, couples, and extended families have also included the decision to raise children and further create families of choice. Queers choosing children runs counter to some Christian theological and cultural notions of families. However, many Queers are rearing children in a variety of circumstances and through a variety of means. Children are often conceived or adopted after Queers have come out. This forces us to

---

*Not all erotic relationships are pair-bonded, monogamous relationships. I believe that we have to escape the tyranny of normativity even within the queer community. What may be normative for myself in a paired-bonded relationship is not necessarily normative for other queer folks. Nontraditional erotic relationships would include relationships such as triadic and quadratic, two bisexual couples who have formed an erotic household, or erotic monastic communities. Theoretically, I have no difficulty with blessing such unions. In practice, I have yet to be asked to bless such a non-pair-bonded relationship.

reexamine the assumptions of Queer identity with actual procreative practice. This reconciliation of identity with procreativity challenges the assumptions of those heterosexuals who claim procreative privileges for themselves and attack Queers for nonproductive hedonism. *Sexual pleasure and procreativity are neither exclusive to one another nor exclusively heterosexual.*

Many gays, lesbians, and bisexuals have custody or share custody of their own children through a former heterosexual marriage. Estimations of lesbian parents range between 1 and 5 million, and the estimations of gay parents range from 1 to 3 million.[14] The American Bar Association estimates that there are 8 to 10 million daughters and sons of lesbian and gay parents.[15]

We have no statistics on bisexual and transgendered families. Transsexuals have often lost their parental custody or coparenting rights in the process of their gender transformation. There are also many lesbian and gay parents who have lost custodial rights to their children. Frequently, two lesbians, who had previously married, have joint custody of their children. A gay parent may share joint custody of his children with his former wife. One partner of a same-sex couple often becomes a coparent to the children of her or his spouse. Sexual procreativity is shared in these parental and coparental families.

John Mollenkopf, a professor of political science at City University of New York analyzed the data from the 1990 census in New York City. The most interesting statistics were that 30 percent of lesbian households had children present, compared with 33 percent of male-headed households (married and unmarried opposite-sex partners). In the same study, 10 percent of gay male households had children.[16] This study undermines the propaganda that gays and lesbians who rear children are rare. It appears from this and other studies that gay and lesbian families in fact are rearing children. Almost the same proportion of lesbian families are rearing children as heterosexual families in New York City. I suspect that this same proportion is also true in other urban areas.

Gays, lesbians, and bisexuals are as capable of procreation as heterosexuals, and many individual and coupled Queers choose to have children. To procreate, some lesbians have sought out gay men who were prepared to be coparents. A number of procreative strategies have been adopted by Queers to raise children and to create families outside the narrow definition of traditional family. It is what the Christian tradition has identified as procreation and wrongfully claims for the nuclear family alone. This decision for procreativity extends the love boundaries of singles, couples, and extended families to include children.

Queers do not undertake procreative strategies unless they really want children and are committed to rearing them. There are no accidental children. Some singles, couples, and extended families have adopted procreative strategies of producing children through reproductive methods such as artificial insemination, invitro fertilization, surrogate motherhood, or sexual intercourse. Most of these strategies challenge conventional understanding of producing offspring. Some lesbians have become parents through artificial insemination, while female or lesbian friends have willingly become artificially inseminated with the sperm of gay singles or couples to produce their children. Sometimes individuals and couples form a household in which to raise children. I know two gay lovers and two lesbian lovers who have had their first daughter through artificial insemination. They share custody and responsibility for the rearing of their daughter within two adjacent households. Some bisexuals have engaged in sexual intercourse to produce children. Parents and surrogate parents form extended families involved in the raising of the children.

Queers may choose an alternative procreative strategy by becoming foster parents, while others have adopted the so-called throwaway children of our society: crack-addicted children, HIV-positive babies, mentally or physically challenged children, children of color, and third-world children. Individual, coupled, and extended families of all sorts have initially involved themselves in foster care and then decided to adopt children. Often adoptions are interracial, adding further social complications. Many white parents of black children include friends of color as extended families to preserve the racial and cultural heritage of their adopted children.

I know of two former Catholic religious men who have formed a communal family with two lesbian lovers concerning the adoption of several African-American children. They have to maintain a low profile because the state adoption laws deny gays and lesbians the right to adopt children. As a Christian minister, I would not hesitate to bless the union of this communal family. This procreative family reflects the inclusive families of God's reign.

Adoption and foster care provide homes for many children who do not have parents willing or able to raise them. I am aware of a lesbian couple who has adopted several severely physically challenged children given up and institutionalized by their families of origin. No one else wanted the disabled children, and this lesbian couple has given them a home and tremendous love. Such examples are far less visible in states that have restricted the opportunities for Queers to provide foster or adoptive homes. The ones who are hurt by these laws are the children.

To adopt, some Queers are compelled to take a low profile even within the Queer community. *The desire for children is stronger than active and visible involvement within the Queer community.* Some gays and lesbians have legally married persons of the opposite sex to adopt children and create extended families. What these individuals and couples have consciously created are homes where children can share the benefit of their love and nurturing. These are loving families of choice.

Queer couples fall in the category of "families of choice" but often participate in the other forms of families previously listed. They remain in partnership through dedication, mutuality, love, and commitment, despite social adversity and cultural pressures to deny their love.

There are no legal or ecclesial bonds to hold Queer couples together, only the daily commitment or the loving choice to stay together. Same-sex couples, like all couples, grow as they work to sustain intimacy, honesty, and open communication.

Fundamentalist Christians and the law have raised questions about whether a child's best interest is served by allowing her or him to be reared by Queer parents. Queer parents, however, differ little from their heterosexual counterparts. Queer parents are as capable of being good parents as heterosexual couples. The sexual orientation of the parents has nothing to do with the orientation, welfare, or development of children. Charlotte Patterson concluded from the summary results of 30 different studies on the children of gays and lesbians that no evidence exists "to suggest that psychological development among children of gay men or lesbians is compromised in any respect relative to studies among the offspring of heterosexual parents."[17] The sexual orientation of the parents has no adverse effect on the psychological and moral development of children. The models of equality between same-sex partners may well be conducive to the development of healthy models of parenting and gender equality.

Perhaps it is easier to recognize the procreativity of families with children and less so with other familial structures. I strongly maintain that families have the right to define themselves. Families have the right to define themselves as families whether there are children involved or not. The notion that there is any one correct form of family must be abandoned, even by Queers, or we run the risk of repeating the violence of compulsory heterosexuality and traditional family values under new rubrics. The kinds of families that queers create are as varied as the kinds of individuals that compose them.[18] A family is no less a family because it does not have the traditional structure of a family.

Friendship serves as the primary paradigm for understanding individual, coupled, and extended relationships. When asked who belongs to their families, Queers often list lovers first, sometimes ex-lovers, certainly friends, and biological family members. Family members are people we can "count on." These include friends and biological family members who accept us. Such friendships take on the roles often provided by biological families. Friendships serve as sources for various kinds of social and emotional support, providing Queers with a network of people with whom they can share celebrations, holidays, and the important moments of life.

Procreative arrangements can also fall outside of the conventional pair-bonding Queer relationships. Friendships built on equal vulnerability, mutuality, compassion, care, and justice-love are found in AIDS/HIV support groups, twelve-step programs, service organizations, and church and activist groups, among many others. Friendships provide much of the emotional support that used to come from families of origin.

The AIDS pandemic has had a profound impact on the lives of gay, lesbian, bisexual, transgendered persons, and their heterosexual friends. To meet the ravages of HIV, we have developed an ethic of care that embodies values associated with family. When both my lover of sixteen years and my brother died on the same day, my friends were there for me. They completely took care of my lover's funeral and reception following the burial service. Throughout that summer, I was numb from grief over the loss of Frank.

I remember that I wanted to become HIV positive and did not care much about living. My friends helped me through my grieving and survivor's guilt, providing me with a safe space to grieve and rebuild my life. Frank's biological relations took his body and buried him in a family plot without acknowledging his 16-year spousal relationship with me. Frank and I had spoken about the final disposition of his body at death, and I acquiesced to the wishes of his father and mother to bury him in a family plot. I clearly understood that I would not be buried with Frank but that the headstone would spell out our spousal relationship. I had celebrated the holidays with his family of origin for eight years and was welcomed in all family gatherings. I had mistakenly understood myself to be part of their family.

Death and grief do strange things to families, and Frank's death from AIDS affected his family of origin's relationship to his family of choice. They abruptly severed all relationship with me, effaced his spousal relationship on the burial headstone, and replaced it solely with his family of origin. The final painful erasure of our covenanted relationship was underscored in the quilt panel that Frank's mother had designed and assembled. All his relatives, including the names of the divorced spouses of his siblings, were included on the quilt panel. There was no mention of me, his life-partner. The erasure of our relationship was then complete.

When I met David, my present life-partner, he further assisted me through the grieving process. One of the extraordinary qualities about David is his loving ability to give me the space to continue to love Frank and to love him as well. One of the first things that David did as we became serious was to visit Frank's gravesite by himself and to speak with him in prayer. He has not expressed the slightest jealousy, never objecting to either pictures of Frank or to my feelings. David's love has been an extraordinary gift of inclusive love. He has, in fact, encouraged me to create a quilt panel memorializing Frank's family of choice, and I completed the quilt in anticipation of the full display of the quilt in Washington, DC, in 1996. Frank and David have taught me the depth and inclusivity of love, and the procreativity of our love has empowered me as a priest-lover. Sexual passion and compassion are procreatively inter-related. My commitment to compassion and justice are expressed in my teaching, activism, and ministry.

Don't let Christian theocrats claim procreativity only for them-selves. Our diverse relationships can be procreative, and we should claim that truth with equal rights and rites, just as heterosexuals do.

Everyone has the right to create a family form that fits her or his needs to realize the human potential for love in nonoppressive relationships. Everyone has the right to define significant relation-ships and decide who matters and counts as family.

NOTES

1. Dennis Altman. *Coming Out in the Seventies.* Sydney: Wild & Wooley, 1979, p. 47.

2. Michel Foucault's interview with James O'Higgins. Reprinted as, "Sexual Choice: Sexual Act: Foucault and Homosexuality." In Lawrence D. Kritzman (Ed.), *Michel Foucault: Politics, Philosophy, Culture, Interviews and Other Writings, 1977-1984.* New York: Routlege, 1988, p. 301.

3. The Friends of Families. *The 1982 Bill of Right of Rights for Families.* Oakland, CA.

4. Robert Goss. *Jesus ACTED UP: A Gay and Lesbian Manifesto.* HarperSanFrancisco, 1993, pp. 136–138.

5. Kath Weston. *Families We Choose: Lesbians, Gays, Kinship.* New York: Columbia University, 1991, p. 208.

6. Margaret Cruikshank. *The Gay and Lesbian Liberation Movement.* New York: Routledge, Chapman & Hall, p. 81

7. L. William Countryman. *Dirt, Greed, & Sex.* Philadelphia: Fortress Press, 1988, pp. 147–167.

8. Countryman, p. 181.

9. Dorothee Soelle. *To Work and to Love: A Theology of Creation.* Philadelphia: Fortress Press, 1984, p. 133.

10. Thomas E. Schmidt. *Straight or Narrow.* Downers Grove, IL: InterVarsity Press, 1995, p. 51

11. Andre Guindon speaks of the sexual fecundity of queer relationships. Andre Guindon. *The Sexual Creators: An Ethical Proposal for Concerned Christians.* New York: University of America Press, 1986, pp. 63–83 and 167–179. See also Robert Goss. "Challenging Procreative Privilege: Equal Rites." *Theology and Sexuality,* 4, 1996, pp. 32-54.

12. Nancy Wilson. *Our Tribe: Queer Folks, God, Jesus and the Bible.* Harper-SanFrancisco, 1995; Eric Rofes. *Reviving Our Tribe.* The Haworth Press, Inc., 1995.

13. Weston, p. 212.

14. Charlotte Patterson. "Children of Lesbian and Gay Parents." *Child Development.* 63(5), October 1992: p. 1026.

15. Cited in a pamphlet published by COLAGE (Children of Lesbians and Gays Everywhere), San Francisco.

16. Jonathan Mandell. "Gay Couples—The Changing Face of New York—Higher Incomes, Better Educated," *New York Newsday.* June 22, 1995, A1, City Section; "Gay Couples—The Changing Face of New York—Gays in Mainstream—Same-Sex Couples Find Home in NYC Census Data," *New York Newsday.* June 22, 1995, A7, City Section.

17. Patterson, p. 1036.

18. See Laura Benkov. *Reinventing the Family: Lesbian and Gay Parents.* New York: Crown Publishing: 1994.

Chapter 2

Queer Culture and Sexuality as a Virtue of Hospitality

Nancy L. Wilson

I came to believe, early on, that the sin of Sodom and Gomorrah was not homosexuality, but inhospitality. I believed that for a long time, until I came to the conclusion that inhospitality was much too mild and euphemistic a word for the violence of Sodom and Gomorrah. I now believe that the sin of Sodom and Gomorrah (like the sin of Gibeah in Judges 19) was ethnic and sexual violence, not inhospitality (as if no one offered the sojourners adequate refreshment).

The time has come, and is in fact overdue, for lesbians, gays, and all Queer folk to dare to move beyond the defensive and to theologize about our struggles and gifts. As an amateur theologian (in the proudest sense of the word) and "Queer millennialist," I believe it is my own peculiar task to follow theological hunches and make suggestions that may either inspire or enrage the professionals. After all the changing movements, fads, and labels (with which, as a full-time pastor, I cannot hope to stay "current"), I've settled on a method of "theological free-association." The following is my attempt to free-associate on the topic of Queer culture and sexuality as a virtue of hospitality.

But first, a story. The starting place of Queer theology is always the *sitz en leben* (the real situation) of our exclusion. On the way to Easter morning services at the Metropolitan Community Church (MCC) of Los Angeles, a church with a special outreach to gays and lesbians, two young boys from the church were riding in the back seat of my car. It is always fascinating to me to try to learn what kids in MCC are learning about God, community, and theology.

One boy was complaining about two kids at MCC's Sunday school, whose bad behavior challenged everyone when they showed up. One child remarked, "I hope they don't show up for the Easter egg hunt. They'll ruin it." To which the other said, "But, it's kinda like communion, you know, everyone is welcome." To which the first child replied, "Communion's one thing, but the Easter egg hunt, too???"

The definition of Queer I want to use comes from several sources: my friends who developed the politics of Queer Nation and Judy Grahn, author of *Another Mother Tongue: Gay Words, Gay Worlds* (Boston, Beacon Press, 1984). I understand Queer to be an inclusive term and a radical political term. It turns the insulting epithet on its ear and includes gays, lesbians, bisexuals, transgendered persons, and all who identify with us politically and culturally. Artists are very frequently Queer, or outside of traditional class structures. Judy Grahn calls such people *transpeople*, and her definition, for me, is the equivalent of "Queer."

Because Queer people are an eclectic tribe, or tribes, it is difficult to get at anything called *Queer culture* and sexuality. However, I do believe that our culture (art; politics; institutions; writings; lifestyles; and ways of being, organizing, and forming relationships and extended families) is very intertwined with our long history of being sexual outlaws in the dominant culture.

There were two primary locations of Queer culture. There has always been the culture of flamboyance: the "streets," Queer culture of the bars and clubs, the drag queens, the butch dykes—in other words, the more marginalized culture of resistance. This was the cultural milieu of the Stonewall Rebellion.

The other side of Queer culture has been the closet—a culture of code words and private, separate social lives, which only occasionally intersected with the street culture. This is probably a function of class as much as anything else. Those with money and power could create private environments and elaborate means of "protection" to insulate themselves from the consequences of breaking the law or flaunting social mores. Despite the rumors that may circulate, we mostly learn about the Queer sexuality of the wealthy and famous when they die. As more of us come out, these two cultures meet, clash, and influence each other.

Virtue is a fascinating word, which is still understood in the parlance of Catholic moral theology, but which has gone out of fashion. It is a little bit anachronistic, conjuring up, for me at least, notions of virginity and purity, even to the point of self-righteousness. It's quite a tight-assed word, actually!

The dictionary offers a far different definition, however. A virtue can be defined as "a particular moral excellence." Its root (the Latin *virtus*, meaning "power") is the same root as for "virile" (the Latin *vir*, meaning "manly"), and it is a synonym for "power, potency, and effective force." *The word virtue then is actually a very butch word!* I am especially attracted to the phrase "a particular moral excellence." Is it possible that our tribes are endowed with any particular moral excellence?

What would it mean for those labeled "Queer," who are considered by many to be *a priori* morally beyond the pale and beyond redemption, to be possessed of a "particular moral excellence?" Moral despair is a terrible killer of our Queer communities. If one is incapable of moral virtue, then one need not bother to try to live in a way that honors one's life, neighbor, or creation. All attempts to live in a healthy, sane manner are futile; all self-improvement and all striving to be good is in vain.

Many Queer folk experience this moral despair as a doorway to all kinds of hells: as the reason not to recover from addictions, as the reason to engage in self-destructive behaviors, as the door to self-hating and all that results from it, as the reason not to pray or work for healing, and as an excuse not to vote or to give and receive love.

Nevertheless, most Queer folks manage profound moral survival, either by concluding (quite rightly) that the whole world is wrong about us, and that moral striving, though useless in terms of what the world might think of us, is still a worthwhile endeavor for a greater audience or by creating very private, almost secret moral zones, rules, and folkways.

A few examples come to mind. When I came out in the early 1970s, it was a Queer moral certainty that you didn't "out" anyone. To do so was to risk exile from the community. The only person I ever had to exclude from an MCC worship service was a deeply disturbed, fanatically religious gay man who attended MCC Boston. He was very verbal at community prayer time and had two academic degrees, including a theological degree from a respectable institution. He was severely disturbed and paranoid.

In addition, he liked to pick up young men at church; take them home and have sex with them; and then engage in a ritual of prayer, repentance, and rebuking in which he verbally threatened his partner. He would find out where the person worked, call their place of employment the next day, and "out" them.

It was not his promiscuous sexual behavior or even his sexual exploitation of young newcomers that morally shocked us; after all why would it have, two decades ago? It was the betrayal of the precious value of the mutually held secret and the putting of others' livelihoods in jeopardy that disrupted the congregation. These were the moral boundaries that could not be crossed. I got a restraining order against him, and it broke my heart because he could not and would not be helped. To exclude anyone from the one and only church in those days that offered shelter to Queers was excruciatingly painful to me. We had tried warning all newcomers (not a very thrilling way to be welcomed to a new church!), but found it didn't work.

Also, there were moral codes and strivings in the bars and clubs—drag show benefits for children, such as "Toys for Tots," many decades before AIDS. There was often almost a desperate attempt to be "community-minded" as hats were passed for partners who were in jail and for those who had lost a job, home, or family. Those tacky bars and clubs were often the only home many people had. Those were sacred spaces, to be kept inviolate. At the bar, there were pecking orders and mentors, as well as people who would, without knowing your last name, or your real name, take you to their homes, feed you, help you get a job, lend you a couple of bucks, and help you get a date. All this they did with no guarantee (in fact, just the opposite) that heaven was their sure reward. *This was virtue for its own sake, in the context of a community of mostly kind strangers.*

When my friend Craig was dying in a convalescent-home-turned-AIDS hospice (at least in the west wing), I saw his stark reliance on this particular moral excellence. The convalescent home found itself needing to hire more gay, lesbian, and Queer nurses and aides for the AIDS wing. Craig told me that it was only the Queer nurses and staff that he didn't give a "hard time to." When a lesbian or gay nurse or aide walked in the room, he relaxed visibly. He knew that not only would they not be indifferent to his pain, but also they would go the extra mile. They would treat him like a brother; they would get him to laugh or to sit up in bed. They'd take a minute to brush his hair, fix his glasses, make him smile, bring him comfort, or tease him. Everyone else frightened him because he had come to believe that they were under no moral obligation to treat him humanely.

I've seen this over and over again in hospitals where a nurse, doctor, or aide would bop in and out, and the hospitalized MCC member would brighten up and let me know that he or she was "family," meaning Queer.

"Hospitality" is also a complex word. I came to know it most in relationship to its negative version, "inhospitality." Since first reading D.S. Bailey's *Homosexuality and the Western Christian Tradition* (Hamdon, CT, Anchor Books, 1975), I came to believe, early on, that the sin of Sodom and Gomorrah was not homosexuality, but inhospitality. I believed that for a long time, until I came to the conclusion that "inhospitality" was much too mild and euphemistic a word for the violence of Sodom and Gomorrah. I now believe that the sin of Sodom and Gomorrah (like the sin of Gibeah in Judges 19) was ethnic and sexual violence, not inhospitality (as if no one offered the sojourners adequate refreshment).

The word *hospitality* or *hospitable* comes from the root word *host* and is related to *hospice* and *hospital*. I am particularly interested in the term *hospice* (where I've spent a fair amount of time in the last ten years). The dictionary defines a hospice as a shelter or rest for pilgrims, strangers, or the terminally ill, often run by a religious order. *Hospitality,* a derivative, is the art of practice of treating guests or strangers warmly.

Hospitality, we learned in studying the Hebrew Scriptures in seminary, was a highly prized virtue of the desert culture. It was a moral imperative in a climate and culture that included travelers and nomads and where isolation and great distances between cities and villages limited one's options. One had to be sure that if shelter, food, or drink was necessary, one could approach a stranger, or a strange village and not be violated, exploited, or refused. It was a matter of life and death.

I was fascinated that the definition of hospice was first of a shelter for pilgrims and strangers and only later came to be used for a place of decent dying. The dying are certainly pilgrims, spiritually and physically.

The definition of religious orders providing refuge for weary travelers is obviously a medieval derivation. I am reminded of John Boswell's book, *The Kindness of Strangers* (New York, Vintage Books, 1990), in which he explores the monasteries and convents of medieval Europe. He develops a haunting hypothesis that the often very gay and lesbian communities of brothers and sisters actually took in and raised many abandoned children in an age that knew no artificial contraception and little about abortion or adoption. He hypothesizes that they actually saved and raised hundreds of thousands of children in massive unsung heroic efforts.

I think of the hospices now staffed mostly by Queer folk who take in abandoned and dying AIDS patients. In many ways, the dying are as vulnerable as children and have become our spiritual and moral children. Also, in the midst of all the dying in our Queer communities, there has been an actual baby boom, which includes the adoption of many abandoned and medically and socially fragile children. The names of the institutions may have changed but not the identity of the workers.

It seems as though the Queer folk of the Middle Ages, including the artists, by the way, made their home in the church, and in turn gave themselves to hospicing. There are still thousands of Queer folks who do this in the Church today, though mostly undercover. More often than not, the Queer tribes have exited the Church, which has proven most inhospitable, even violent.

In *Original Blessing* (Santa Fe, Bear & Co., 1983), Matthew Fox offers a powerful analysis of the differences between creation- and redemption-centered spirituality. He clarified for me that to define the problem is to define its solution. If the problem is sin, as narrowly defined as a condition (acted out) of being morally out of the will of God, then redemption through atonement is the logical solution. John Stott's book, *The Cross of Christ* (Intervarsity, 1988), is the best and most bone-chilling theological description of "the" orthodox view of atonement. I find his view of sin, God, and atonement repulsive, cruel, and highly logically consistent with dominant .

assumptions about sin and God. His view is that God is too perfect and holy to tolerate any sin or evil, that God's wrath had to be satisfied by a blood sacrifice, and that Jesus was pure enough to satisfy and pay the penalty for our sin: "God had to kill Jesus to save me because I'm so wicked."

If the central moral problem is not sin, defined as utter, abject disapproval by God, but is instead a condition of alienation, homelessness, and rejection, then a solution to this human problem (which also has been labeled "sin") might be the process of "at-home-ment." For me, the story of the Prodigal Child (Luke 15) is the quintessential Jesus story of the nature of sin and "at-home-ment." The most compelling and powerful moment in the story occurs while the son is making up his excuse speech, hoping to convince the father to take him in (but only as a servant). The Gospel of Luke (15:21) says that "while he was yet afar off" the father ran to him to embrace him and to welcome him home.

Queer folks have, over time, especially in Western culture, developed a collective separation anxiety and the morbid fear of loss of home, family, religion, nation, and God. We have creatively invented substitutes for all of the above, sometimes to our delight, and sometimes to our destruction.

I believe that God is present in our communities, creating the hope and reality of "at-home-ment." God does this, I believe, as we Queer folks exercise our tribal gifts of hospitality toward and within our own community and in the world.

Many have written and commented on the existence of a Queer sensibility that includes interior decorating and party planning and execution. *One of the methods of providing hospitality is to create environments of beauty, safety, and home. Is there an internal logic to the culturally and spiritually homeless developing skills, over time (passed down through Queer generations) for creating "beautiful homes and gardens?"*

I think of the movie *To Wong Fu, Thanks for Everything, Julie Newman* and the drag queens' gift of decorating and party throwing, while pursuing their mission of intervening in a situation of domestic violence. These queer visitors were meddlers and bringers of cheer, advice, and color to a colorless, despairing, no-account town. They are another version of the Wise Men coming to announce change, redemption, and creation of "at-home-ment." They are not just there for decoration but for a higher purpose.

I am reminded of another friend, Tom, whom I visited a few times in his last days at a hospice near a church. Tom's memorial service was held in the clubhouse of his friend's apartment complex. Present were friends, old and new; family members; and much of the staff of the hotel where he worked as chief concierge for many years. His friends tried to create an elegant party for his memorial service.

Over and over, the same theme repeated itself during the memorial service time of sharing—Tom as an inveterate tour guide, who wanted you to have the best time in his city; the timeless party maker; the one who cheered and encouraged, who made you feel at home. I was especially touched by the heterosexual men and women who, awkwardly at first, not as used to dozens of these memorial services, sobbed and choked as they told their stories. There was a young guitar player whom Tom took under his wing and made feel safe, and there was a young bride who described the amazing surprise bridal shower thrown for her. Tom's generosity and hospitality constituted a particular moral excellence that was unmistakable.

The lesbian women at the California Institute for Women, a correctional facility, who attend Free Spirit MCC* love to have parties often. I'm always touched and amazed at how they put together a "spread" from cheese and crackers spirited away from the lunch line and hidden in their clothing. They are not permitted to bring snacks to the chapel for celebrations. However, on the tenth anniversary of weekly MCC services in that place of despair and alienation that often says, "You can never return home; you don't deserve a home," they managed to sneak in all kinds of treats, bits and pieces, scraps, little napkins and plates, and even a tablecloth. They were proud, and we ate hearty. For just a minute here and there, it was entirely possible to forget where we were.

This does not mean, however, that there is no human or moral evil to contend with. Moral despair in whole groups of people, in fact, is the breeding ground for evil. Also, Queer folks have been

---

*Free Spirit MCC is a church behind prison walls.

encouraged to lie by the dominant culture, and it is lying that also breeds evil (see M. Scott Peck's *People of the Lie* [New York, Simon & Schuster, 1983]) and moral confusion.

What restores human moral agency is not the threat of punishment or guilt but being able to tell the truth and face the consequences (even the unjust ones) and reclaim our full human dignity. This is one of the themes of the movie *Dead Man Walking*. When Matthew Poncelet, murderer and rapist, found "at-home-ment" in Sister Helen's presence, which relentlessly required the truth from him, he found a safe place in which to reclaim his basic human capacity for moral discernment and action. This is the most profound hospitality possible. It is "at-home-ment," which is salvific.

I deal with the idea of an ethic of sexuality in terms of "bodily hospitality" in my book *Our Tribe: Queer Folks, God, Jesus and the Bible* (HarperSanFrancisco, 1995). One reviewer called this a "deliciously wicked" theological idea. I have to guess what he meant by that. I can only assume that the concept of sexuality at its best, being conceived of as bodily hospitality, was interpreted by him to mean that I was proposing no limits on sexual activity or that it was such a positive image of sexual relations that it invited him or others to consider all sexual activity as moral or good, and that that was a "deliciously wicked" (permissive?) idea.

His comment certainly spoke to me of the depth to which our ethicizing about sexuality, for some people, has to be in the context of moral limits, judgment, rules (to minimize the bad stuff!), or the mob is incomplete somehow. As if celebration and permissiveness (in an age of AIDS, especially) are in themselves "deliciously wicked."

I think that there is a tremendous tension in Queer communities about how to approach sexual ethics at all. And here, when I say "Queer," I include feminists. I think there are two "poles of values" in dynamic tension about how to theologize and ethicize about sexuality.

The first I would identify around the pole of safety. Marie Fortune's book, *Love Does No Harm* (New York: Continuum, 1995), and the entire movement for AIDS-based safer sex come to mind. Here the ethic is rooted in the imperative to do no harm and to minimize violence and disease. It seeks to identify and label sexual relating that is exploitive, addictive, or violent in the broadest sense, and to exclude it as morally inferior. This is a popular position of many second-wave feminists who categorically view all "pornography" as inherently immoral, exploitive, and antifemale. Similarly, feminists, lesbian and straight, see all forms of sadomasochism (even those that are highly monitored, consensual, and experienced as sexual play) as inherently violent and exploitive as well.

In drawing a circle of containment around any sexual relation that is labeled unsafe, it is harder to focus on and define the essential goodness of sexuality. Perhaps it is simply a matter of emphasis. *Queer communities have had to do a lot more analyzing about what is safe—much more than the dominant culture, which assumes that what is legal, sanctioned, and approved is automatically safe, healthy, and holy (a very bad assumption, by the way).*

But is safety sexy? And does it need to be? Safe sex ads and videos have bombarded gay men ad nauseam, with indoctrination that assures them that safe sex is sexy. It is, it can be, it must be, and it will be. Each generation of gay men, it seems, struggles to be convinced. And women, lesbian or straight, are less the targets of such indoctrination, mostly I fear, because it doesn't serve men's needs for women to be overly concerned about their safety. We are encouraged to be objects of sexiness (whether straight, lesbian, or bisexual) and accessible to men, no matter what. Encouraging women to be safe will not achieve this goal.

The other "pole of value," sometimes in tension with the value of safety, is freedom and celebration. This is what I believe the reviewer perceived as "deliciously wicked" in a Christian ethical context. One can be free and celebrate sexuality hedonistically, for the intrinsic value of pleasure in and of itself. To do so means believing that the freedom to share one's body sexually is an intrinsic right, and the purpose need not be greater (morally or otherwise) than the sheer, singular value of pleasure.

How much does that singular value of pleasure need to be modified by safety? I remember a haunting conversation at the deathbed of a young man dying of AIDS. I was called to be with him in his dying for six weeks or so. I was called because he was terrified of dying and terrified of God. He grew up in a religious home. At age 14, when his mother died, his father began a reign of violent terror on him. He ran away from home and never returned. He survived on the streets any way he could. He developed certain patterns in his sexuality, which included some mild forms of sadomasochism and liberal drug use. He became financially successful, had good jobs, and used his exquisite good looks to land many modeling jobs.

He managed to get clean and sober, but not before he contracted HIV. Even after sobriety, he could not modify his sexual behavior consistently. One day, he trembled as he told me how riddled with guilt he was, that he had killed himself, and that he was afraid he could not be forgiven by God. He told me that he loved "wild sex" and even now missed it terribly. For him "wild sex" meant unsafe sex, unfettered by condoms or other sexual boundaries. Even as he spoke to me from a body racked with pain, nearly a skeleton, part of him reveled in the memory of that pleasure, and part of him writhed in pain of the guilt of exchanging life (safety) for pleasure.

I was so aware of how complex this was—how all his early sexual cuing was tied to his mother's loss, his father's abuse and sadism, and his plunge into the culture of street survival sex. I'm not sure that he ever accepted forgiveness for neglecting his own safety. His dying attachment to the pleasure, which hastened his death, haunts me in ways I have not yet resolved.

I still think that Christians could spend centuries recovering the intrinsic goodness of God's creation of the gift of sexuality and sexual pleasure without overdoing it. It is the "repression" that I believe leads to "obsession." The obsession with sex in our culture is so riddled with reactivity to repression that it is really not sexy at all. It is cartoonish, garish, vile, and often more repelling than attracting. How long will it take us to get off the repression-obsession sexual merry-go-round and embrace sexual pleasure as a part of healthy, joyful living.

W.H. Auden did say, "As a rule, it is the pleasure-haters who were unjust." They were also, as a rule, Christian. Pleasure-hating is not a virtue, it is not moral excellence, and it shrivels and distorts the human spirit. It ultimately kills.

Roman Catholic ethicist Dan Maguire said (at an MCC conference) that he thought the Church should take a long break (a century?) from making any "pelvic pronouncements" or ethicizing or theologizing below the waist. He insisted that the institutional Church is not credible or competent to do anything useful in terms of sexuality, in view of its refusal both to encourage safety and to celebrate freedom.

I think that the concept of sexuality as bodily hospitality has the potential to reconcile the "poles of value" of safety and celebration; that is, in creating a theology of bodily "at-home-ment," in which we view sexuality as one way we share the home of our bodies, emotions, and passions with others.

If hospitality is the virtue, the "particular moral excellence" of treating guests or strangers warmly, how might "bodily hospitality" be a reconciling ethical starting place for human sexual relating? If my body is my physical home, I am challenged to view my body in terms of "at-home-ment." My body as the "temple of my own being and of God's presence within me. To relate sexually is to invite another into my body/home/space. To treat others "warmly" in my sexual relating, to be hospitable, might begin to express the poles of value of safety and freedom andcelebration.

For most of us, this means continuous efforts at "home improvement"—taking care of our bodies and our mental and spiritual health; understanding the deep and painful forces that can lead to poor judgment, lack of impulse control, or addiction; or understanding the equally tragic forces that lead to isolation, deprivation, loneliness, and despair—risking the wrong thing or not risking the right thing enough.

Why is it that some of us so easily share our bodies with strangers in a risky manner, when we would never offer them the keys to our car or house? How many times have we turned away from love, intimacy, and pleasure, feeling unworthy, frightened, and unable to believe or trust that sexual pleasure, play, or intimacy is possible or worth the risk? Inviting someone into our home always means risks, negotiating boundaries, and mutual commitment in turn for certain gains. This is just as true for sexual relating.

The Church, spiritual home for Christians, is Christ's body. Jesus, I believe, exercised and exercises bodily hospitality toward us. The image is powerful and unequivocal. We are participants, included, incarnated, and incorporated in Christ's body. In MCC we practice "open communion," choosing the value of inclusivity over exclusivity. It means that we open Christ's body to newcomers, strangers, and those who are even ambivalent spiritually, teetering on the edge, uncertain. It is our prayer that the invitation, itself, and the Holy Spirit will heal the spiritually wounded and wavering. By incarnating a Christ with permeable boundaries, we risk, I suppose, many things. But we affirm that Christ in us is clear and strong enough to withstand the fuzziness of fewer rules and barriers. Safety and freedom are twin issues that challenge our spiritual body.

How is the invitation to church, to communion, to be included in Christ's body, accomplished with the virtue of hospitality? Is the symbolic invitation of Christ into one's body another communal metaphor for hospitality? Is the test of our authenticity as Christ's Church the way we warmly include guests and strangers?

The pleasure of the practice of bodily hospitality of communion in MCC is one of the great joys of my life. It may be the primary gift of queers to the Church—a "particular moral excellence" borne of our experience of *exclusion* and one that drives us to *include* with a vengeance (even at Easter egg hunts with unruly children). Perhaps our interpretation helps create the beloved community that Christ lived, died, and rose to bring.

Chapter 3

The Concubine and the Eunuch
Queering Up the Breeder's Bible

Victoria S. Kolakowski

I find it particularly ironic that the most compelling scriptural argument for gay and lesbian affirmation in the Christian scriptures may come from the teachings about the transgendered eunuchs, since transgendered people are second-class citizens in the Queer Christian community.

It was when I had first begun associating with gay and lesbian political activists (nobody would dare identify as bisexual or transgendered) after coming out in New Orleans in 1989, that I first heard the word *oppressed* used to describe us. I felt very uncomfortable with the word because it sounded so, well, politically correct, and it seemed excessive. After all, when I thought about oppression, I thought about things like apartheid, segregation, Jim Crow laws, Communist rule behind the Iron Curtain, or life in Nazi Germany. If nothing else, I was afraid that we would seem as though we were blowing things out of proportion. I didn't want to be written off by potentially supportive, mainstream, straight, white folk. Even more so, I didn't want us to offend those who had been "truly" oppressed, such as people of color, the survivors of Auschwitz, or others who might feel that we were trivializing their "legitimate" oppression.

As time went by, and I worked extensively in politics and with spirituality, I came to understand that it was *me* who was doing the trivializing, for the word *oppress* literally means "to govern harshly; keep down unjustly or by cruelty."[1] It also means "to weigh down." Whether I wanted to acknowledge it or not, that was something that was happening to me. I have lived my entire life in a society that trivializes my relationships and is in collective denial over the widespread discrimination and violence against gay, lesbian, bisexual, and transgendered people. This is a form of psychic and spiritual cruelty that pressures us into silence and deceit— Don't Ask; Don't Tell.

Thus, I have learned that it is in the areas of our self-identity and self-worth that we gay, lesbian, bisexual, and transgendered people are subject to the most cruelty. Psychologically and spiritually, we are weighed down, and often crushed. What can be more cruel than to teach children as they are growing up that they are hated by their creator? Queer children are told that their natural urges to love and be loved are not merely undesirable or inappropriate, but that they are *evil* and that they will result in eternal punishment. This is horrible and cruel. To plant in a young child's mind the seeds of her or his own self-hatred is not new; it is an experience that African Americans and other people of color have faced in the United States since its founding. However, we still struggle to acknowledge this oppression to ourselves, and the collective denial barely has been touched.

I am not saying that this is some sort of organized conspiracy of bigots intent on oppressing us. *I believe that the majority of this burdening comes not from individual, conscious decision making but rather from social institutions, customs, and structures that are organized in such a way that by their very nature they are oppressive to us.*

For many, perhaps most, of us living in the United States and other Western countries, the primary social institutions that define our individual and collective spirituality are the Judeo-Christian religions and their scriptures. Because of that, I think it is important for all gay, lesbian, bisexual, and transgendered people to learn about how and why these religions and scriptures have oppressed us and to identify the traditions within those groups and texts that are positive and support us. For those of us who remain within the broad boundaries of those religions, this can be personally satisfying and can lead to increased self-esteem. However, for all of us, no matter what our own personal spirituality is, this can provide both a new vision for how we look at ourselves and a new message that we can communicate to those people who want to be supportive and yet believe that their religion condemns us.

These social institutions are grounded in a history that goes back millennia. For those of us who participate in the Judeo-Christian traditions, beliefs and customs are supported by our interpretation of texts that were written over a period lasting 1,000 years, the most recent being almost 2,000 years old. These texts are written with all sorts of unstated assumptions about the world, many of which may seem alien to us.

The oldest references to social institutions and relationships in the Judeo-Christian tradition are found in the Hebrew Scriptures, known to Christians as the Old Testament. Some of these appear to be common today, such as marriage and the relationships between parents and children. Others, such as tribes, concubines, slaves, and eunuchs, seem to be familiar, more so to some of us than others. One of the most important things to understand, though, is that no matter how familiar these relationships may seem to us, they were not really the way we view them now.

For example, marriage was not about romance, and certainly not about a woman's romantic concerns. Marriages were primarily political and economic arrangements, for the most part formally decided by men. In addition, marriages were not just between individuals; they brought individual clans or tribes into relationship with each other.

Raising male children to be men's heirs was central to the family structure. This was more important than just a question of who would inherit the property of a man when he died. In ancient society, family name and honor were very important. This was particularly true of the nomadic ancestors of the Israelites, for whom reputation was probably the only stable thing available when they engaged in commerce. Without male children, a man's name perished, and perhaps the name of the entire clan or tribe might be threatened. Without female children, there would be nobody to marry off to other tribes/families or to do the work of the home. As a result, parenthood and parentage were very important to the preservation of the tribe/family and a man's name. In an age before genetic paternity tests, it was essential that each woman have only one male sexual partner, to ensure that the paternity of any children was accurately known.*

Strict rules existed regarding the control of sexuality (especially female sexuality), which were closely connected to the rules of marriage and inheritance. Marriage and procreation were universally understood duties for both sexes, for both economic and sociopolitical reasons. To violate these rules governing sexuality was more than just a personal affront or private indiscretion. Entire communities could be affected by such violations, since they affected the future heritage of the family and the family's relationship with other families. Hence, the response was often severe. For example, to sleep with the wives and/or the concubines of the king was considered equivalent to usurping the throne.[2] When a woman violated these rules, she was cast out of society, was unable to marry, and hence was usually condemned to a life of prostitution, if she were permitted to live.

Life did not always adhere to this plan for many people, including straight, married people. Sometimes men and women did not have male heirs to inherit their name and property. Suppose this were because the man died before having a son. What would happen to his name? A "rule" was created for just this sort of situation. The widow would marry the most closely related male relative of the deceased man, and the sons of the widow would be considered the sons of the *dead* man, not of the new husband. In this way, the name of the dead man would be preserved. This arrangement is known as a *levirate* marriage.

What if the male relatives didn't want to do this? One biblical story, that of Judah's sons and his daughter-in-law Tamar, explains such a situation:

> But Er, Judah's firstborn, was wicked in the sight of the LORD, and the LORD put him to death. Then Judah said to Onan, "Go in to your brother's wife and perform the duty of a brother-in-law to her; raise up offspring for your brother." But since Onan knew that the offspring would not be his, he spilled

---

*By extension, this speaks to why matriarchies work very well in establishing lineage. You always know who a child's mother is, but you can't always be sure who the father is.

his semen on the ground whenever he went in to his brother's wife, so that he would not give offspring to his brother. What he did was displeasing in the sight of the LORD, and he put him to death also. (Gen 38:7–10 [NRSV])

The moral of this story, obviously, is to do one's duty to keep alive the name of one's deceased brother.* This story has been misinterpreted to become the primary scriptural condemnation of male masturbation, and the practice of ejaculation without insemination has historically been known as *onanism*.

The Book of Ruth offers another story about surrogate fatherhood, in which Ruth marries Boaz, a male relative of her late husband Kilion. The fourth chapter offers a fascinating description of a ceremony for determining who would marry the widow and maintain the name of the deceased man. The ceremony of this story makes explicit the surrogate nature of Ruth's remarriage.**

Both stories show how a fiction was used to maintain the name of deceased men by having the widows remarry other men of the families. These stories demonstrate that marriage is really to the family and not simply to the man himself. They also demonstrate that the traditional notions of marriage were stretched to accommodate unusual situations.

A similar fiction was used when a wife could not bear a child. In most ancient Near East societies, men were allowed to have a secondary wife, called a *concubine,* who functioned at times as a surrogate for the wife (the concubines of Israel were likely to have been from a family of lower class, whose families were not worthy of political alliance with that of the man; hence, the secondary

---

*Interestingly, the story goes on to describe how Tamar disguises herself as a prostitute to seduce Judah because he would not marry his remaining son to her, and she bears Judah twin sons. This story, like the story of Ruth, is neither entirely consistent in its application of the rules stated elsewhere in the Torah (Law), the way that it handles the response to Tamar's ploy, nor with the way that the rules came to be applied at later times. This shows that the social rules bent with time to accommodate sociopolitical realities.

**Ruth 4. The response of the women of the town to Ruth and Boaz having a son—"[T]he women living there said, 'Naomi has a son.'" (Ruth 4:17)—suggests that the story recognized an additional type of surrogacy in this story as well.

nature of the marriage). A child of the secondary wife could be considered to be that of the barren woman.

A well-known example of this is seen in the biblical story of Abraham, Sarah, and Hagar.* Sarah was barren, and Hagar gave birth to a son, Ishmael, who was to be considered the son of Sarah. As with most cases of this type, Sarah was of a higher class than Hagar. Some scholars even suggest that Sarah may have been a priestess of a goddess cult.**

So again, it appears that the Bible records that this society created surrogacy forms; that is, legal fictions that included exceptions to the rules, allowing people's needs to be met when circumstances did not quite work as required under the rules, particularly when those fictions served the social purposes underlying the rules. The lines in these cases were blurred, and the hard-and-fast rules were adapted to meet the needs of some rich and powerful members of the community for whom the rules didn't work.

Also during this time, there was a whole class of people who were incapable of bearing children—the eunuchs. The traditional definition of eunuch is a male born without genitals, or a castrated male, and it is clear in the Hebrew Scriptures that such eunuchs were in a terrible position in the society. They were excluded from participating in the religious ritual life of the community. Because they were incapable of having children, they could not continue their name, which we have seen was paramount in ancient society.

Eunuchs were discussed by ancient Jewish, Greek, and Roman writers. Finding references to eunuchs, per se, in the Old Testament is complicated by the ambiguity of the words used for them, since in

---

*Gen. 16 and 21. See particularly verse 2: ". . . and Sarai said to Abram, 'You see that the LORD has prevented me from bearing children; go in to my slave-girl; it may be that *I shall obtain children by her'* " (emphasis added).

**See Savina J. Teubal. *Sarah the Priestess: The First Matriarch of Genesis.* Athens, OH: Swallow Press/Ohio University Press, 1984, and its sequel, *Hagar the Egyptian: The Lost Tradition of the Matriarchs.* San Francisco: Harper & Row, 1990. Racism seems to also be a factor in this story, since Hagar was an Egyptian slave. One might also wonder if racism is a factor in the way that the white, mainstream, middle-class churches have recently promoted the role of Sarah without ever mentioning Hagar, nor for considering the social realities of this story. The classism and racism of the surrogacy relationship continues to this date, as can be seen from any examination of modern surrogacy arrangements.

both Greek and Hebrew the word for eunuch means both *castrated male* and *high government official.** However, despite this association with powerful political position, even the most important eunuchs in the ancient world also were subject to public shame because of their castrated state and inability to procreate.** Sociologists have shown that characteristics considered deviant have a more powerful effect on how one is treated than characteristics considered validating the conventional. Thus, we can reasonably assume that eunuchs must have been more strongly despised than held in high esteem.***

The Israelites had firm rules for ostracizing eunuchs, banning them from participating in the religious (and thereby social) life of the community.**** This is not surprising, for eunuchs are outside the ordinary kinship notions of ancient Palestine, individuals in a world of family and nation.[3] Nevertheless, there are a number of eunuchs in the Old Testament who clearly had important and positive roles.***** The end of the social stigmatization of eunuchs was prophesied in Isaiah:

---

*As an example of this ambiguity, Potiphar, the Egyptian Captain of the Guard (Gen. 37:36), who bought Joseph in slavery, is referred to as a "saris" (Hebrew for eunuch) in both Gen 37:36 and Gen. 39:1, despite the fact that he is best known for his wife's sexual advances toward Joseph. Most modern scholars believe that Potiphar was not a castrated man, although it might well explain his wife's behavior!

**Many ancient writers, including Herodotus, Lucian of Samosata, Petronius, Josephus and Philo, wrote disparagingly about eunuchs. Castration of other humans, particularly young boys, became widespread in the Roman Empire and was eventually (unsuccessfully) banned, punishable by death. Jewish theologians and Scripture also disparaged eunuchs.

***The experience of being both valued for one's contributions while being socially despised is one understood by many of us gay and lesbian people, since certain professions have been stereotypically gay in a society that despises us. Often the same people who don't want us in their churches or for us to marry are proud to have a gay hairdresser or interior designer.

****Deuteronomy states, "No one whose testicles are crushed or whose penis is cut off shall be admitted to the assembly of the Lord" (Dt. 23:1). Leviticus states that a variety of physical deformities, including crushed testicles, were a bar to the priesthood (Lev. 21:16–23).

*****See Nancy Wilson. *Our Tribe: Queer Folks, God, Jesus and the Bible.* HarperSanFrancisco, 1995, pp. 281–285. Also, scholarly arguments have been made that both Daniel and Nehemiah were eunuchs.

> Do not let the foreigner joined to the LORD say, "The LORD
> will surely separate me from his people"; and do not let the
> eunuch say, "I am just a dry tree." For thus says the LORD:
> To the eunuchs who keep my Sabbaths, who choose the things
> that please me and hold fast my covenant, I will give, in my
> house and within my walls, a monument and a name better
> than sons and daughters; I will give them an everlasting name
> that shall not be cut off. (Isaiah 56:3–5)

The connection between eunuchs and barrenness is made particularly clear in this passage. The continuation of a man's name served
as a monument to him. This prophecy promised the eunuchs a
restoration to the social benefits of fathering children, notwithstanding the eunuch's physical incapacity to do so. Nevertheless, this
apparently was viewed as being a promise for the distant future, and
therefore this prophecy appears to have had little effect on the
treatment of eunuchs under the law in postexilic Judea.*

Eunuchs had a different religious position in some other parts of
the ancient Greek and Roman worlds. There were cults in Asia
Minor with priests who were castrated men, often castrated by their
own hand. The best known example of this is the cult of Cybele,
centered at Galatia; but similar practices were found in the cults of
Attis and Artemis of Ephesus. These eunuch-priests were known as
bacheloi or *galloi,* and held positions of high honor. However, they
were actually more priestesses than priests in the roles that they
filled.

Eunuchs were viewed as being of ambiguous gender in the
ancient Greek and Roman worlds outside of Palestine. For example,
in the Cybele cult, the eunuch's service was in the role of a priestess. In addition, eunuchs lacking secondary sexual characteristics,
such as a beard, were often used for pederastic. Others, however,
were feminized, and they chose to live their lives as women.
Although situations differed, it is clear that eunuchs fell within the
sexual category that we would today broadly call *transgendered,*

---

*Horner suggests that this prophecy was included because there was a concern
among the exiles in Babylon for some among their number who had become
eunuchs and thus excluded from the community. Tom Horner. *Jonathan Loved
David*. Philadelphia: Westminster Press, 1978, pp. 82–83.

and many would be considered transsexual. *As a result, many of my transgendered sisters look to the ancient eunuchs for affirmation of our history and spirituality.* Some scholars believe that the term eunuch was used to identify more people than just castrated men. Ancient rabbis referred to those made eunuchs by men as well as those made eunuchs by birth, which seems to have included men who were genitally deformed or physically incapable of procreation. Further, some scholars believe that the term eunuch was used as a derogatory slang word for men who did not have children, and that the word was therefore one term used for gay men who refused to marry women.* Therefore, references to eunuchs should have special meaning for gay men. I would like to point out, however, that this is a figurative connection, and that the primary connection is to the *transgendered person* of the ancient world, that is, the eunuch. *It is in the commonality of the two groups, our common Queerness, our breaking of the procreative and gender stereotypes of the society, our unique ability to separate our sexuality from procreation, that is the issue here.*

It is with this in mind that we should look at the first of two references to eunuchs in the Christian Scriptures, or the New Testament. The first is found in Matthew 19:12: "For there are eunuchs who have been so from birth, and there are eunuchs who have been made eunuchs by others, and there are eunuchs who have made themselves eunuchs for the sake of the kingdom of heaven. Let anyone accept this who can." This passage has received a great deal of attention from commentators throughout history and in modern times from Roman Catholic scholars because of its traditional interpretation as a reference to a call for a celibate priesthood, although the only debate has been over who Jesus intended to remain celibate.**

---

*John J. McNeill writes, "The first category—those eunuchs who have been so from birth—is the closest description that we have in the Bible to what we understand today as a homosexual." In *The Church and the Homosexual,* fourth edition. Boston: Beacon Press, 1993, p. 65. See also Nancy L. Wilson. *Our Story Too.* Los Angeles: Universal Fellowship of Metropolitan Community Churches, 1992, pp. 4–6, 8.

**While this has been viewed as a figurative call, some ancient Christians took it literally, including possibly Eusebius, and this became such a problem that the establishment Christian Church eventually decided to excommunicate those who practiced self-castration.

Is this statement about celibacy? I don't think so. Being a eunuch wasn't about not having sex but about not producing offspring. As we all know, one can be quite sexual without having children—all one has to do is abstain from genital-genital, opposite-sex contact. Eunuchs were often sexually active, contrary to modern misunderstandings. So this statement cannot logically be about what we've always been told it is about—the rejection of sexuality.

What does this strange saying really mean? What is clear from the text is that there are three categories of eunuch listed—from birth, made by others, and for the sake of the kingdom of heaven—the first two being the standard categories for eunuchs in rabbinical teachings. The third category is not found in any pre-Christian source and is generally believed, by even the most skeptical scholars, to be original to Jesus.*

It is widely believed by scholars that Jesus, himself, had been derisively called a eunuch, and that it was this charge to which Jesus was responding in this statement. Jesus, as far as is known, never married and did not have any children. As a result, he was considered a procreative deviant, which was considered sociopathic.

But Jesus didn't respond by distancing himself from the eunuchs, the transgendered, and (likely) the gay men of his time, or by making some clear distinction and defining himself as "good" and them as "bad." Instead, he created a third category of the procreatively deviant, those made eunuchs for the sake of the kingdom, which he clearly implies includes himself. The radicalness of this lifestyle choice should not be overlooked or influenced by our modern acceptance that not having children is an acceptable life choice. Jesus' refusal to settle down and marry was undoubtedly more socially deviant than the Greek and Roman practice of marrying and raising a family while having homosexual relationships on the side. By making this statement, Jesus identifies himself boldly with the eunuch, whom his society considered sexually deviant, *Queer.*

I know that many gay and lesbian people dislike using the word *Queer,* but it is entirely appropriate here. I believe that the word

---

*This is likely to be an authentic saying of Jesus because of its novelty, its early origin in Christian writing, and the lack of any imaginable purpose of the saying for the early church, combined with the harshness and shockingness of the imagery.

eunuch, applied to Jesus, was as derogatory and hateful as the word *Queer* is in modern times, and it also meant to include many of the same type of people—the transgendered, the queens, the "out" gay men, and the other sexual minorities of the time. But Jesus took that derogatory slang word thrown at him and proudly claimed it as part of his own identity. This is exactly what modern activists have done with the word *Queer.* Jesus' saying here was an "in-your-face" comeback, and it was so shockingly powerful that his followers remembered it and later wrote it down. We need to proudly acknowledge this and inform our fundamentalist Christian detractors that Jesus was "Queer" in his society's eyes and that he claimed us to be his family.

The second reference to eunuchs in the New Testament, found in Acts 8:26–40, is the story of an encounter between the disciple Philip, and an Ethiopian eunuch. In this story, an unnamed Ethiopian eunuch was traveling on the same road as Philip, reading aloud from a scroll of the Book of Isaiah about "the Suffering Servant." The eunuch asked Philip to help interpret the story. Philip argued that the passage referred to Jesus and told the eunuch the good news about Jesus. The eunuch asked what must be done to be baptized, and then he asked to be baptized in some nearby water. After the baptism, the two went their separate ways.

This is a well-known story about conversion and baptism, particularly popular with American evangelicals because of its power and simplicity as a baptism story, as well as with African Americans because of its empowering vision of a significant black African as a major early Christian convert. Regardless of our vantage point, we can learn a lot by the fact that the major character being baptized is a eunuch; amazingly, a point that these same groups overlook.

What is striking about this story is the apparent nonimportance of the fact that this person is a eunuch. That this eunuch was indeed a castrated man, and not just a high government official, is clear from the text.* Given that a eunuch would be barred from the traditional practice of ancient Judaism, the complete lack of attention to this

---

*First, the eunuch is described as a eunuch and then as treasurer, which is redundant if eunuch is meant simply to refer to a high official. Second, treasurers were often eunuchs. Finally, the treasurer serves the Candace (queen) of Ethiopia, and queens were often served by castrated men.

point is striking; it is a total nonissue. Is this story a sign of the partial fulfillment of the prophecy of Isaiah regarding the inclusion of eunuchs into the religious life of the people?

Some might say that the convert's identity as a eunuch is a nonissue because it wasn't the eunuch's "fault." The eunuch was an "innocent victim" with a physical impairment. If that were the case, then why is there no healing miracle offered in this story? If being a eunuch were considered a physical problem, then why is this the only story in the New Testament where a known physical defect is not cured as part of the absolution from sin and restoration of relationship to God and the people? If being a eunuch were considered only a behavioral or attitudinal problem, then why is there no call to repentance?

The radicalness of this story lies in the fact that the early Christian Church appeared to think that baptizing a eunuch was nothing so important as to be even worth discussing. No moral condemnation is implied. There is the appearance of total acceptance because Jesus spoke about and identified himself as a eunuch for God's reign. In the following centuries, the Christian elite made themselves spiritual eunuchs. Given the transgendered nature of eunuchs and the close association of eunuchs to gay men, this could be an important lesson to the Christian churches that continue to exclude us from their ranks.

I have shown that in ancient Palestine procreation was considered essential to maintaining the family name and integrity, and that the whole society was dependent on rigid gender roles and regulations of women's procreative abilities and human sexuality. At the same time, I have also shown that for certain privileged people, exceptions were permitted. In addition, forms of surrogacy such as the levirate marriage and the bearing of children by a concubine were used to get around the problems. The rigid rules were blurred.

Further, I have shown how the ultimate breakdown of this procreative imperative occurred for a despised class of people, the eunuchs, who actually include the sexual minorities of the ancient Greek and Roman worlds as they knew them. Notwithstanding the diminished status of the eunuchs in the ancient Hebrew Scriptures, there was hope prophesied for eunuchs in the Book of Isaiah. In the Christian tradition, the hope is more strongly realized by Jesus' radical statement of solidarity with eunuchs and the later example of the baptism of the Ethiopian eunuch without comment or qualification.

But where does this leave us today? It leaves us in a more powerful position to go toe-to-toe with those Christians who reject gay and lesbian people or question just what role we are to play both in religious circles and in society as a whole. For if in ancient times the rigid lines around procreation could blur in the light of social reality, and if both Jesus and the early Christian Church had no problem with us, embraced us with open arms, and stood in solidarity with us, who are present-day Christians to do otherwise?

As a lesbian transsexual Christian, these New Testament stories are extremely powerful statements of validation and acceptance from Jesus and the early Christian Church. This is unlike the message that well-meaning gay and lesbian biblical scholars have been sending—that the Christian Scriptures are simply neutral rather than overtly negative about us. I believe they paint a very different picture, one in which there is a voice of specific affirmation of us, one which I am not inventing just to feel accepted. We need to take ownership of this radical message.

These stories also point to something else that is very important to me as a transgendered person. Too often it seems that the mainstream gay and lesbian community has felt that acceptance of transgendered people into this community is one of solidarity with a group, which otherwise has no tie to the community. I have felt that this inclusion is merely a patronizing one of sympathy for other excluded people too powerless and few to even form their own communities. I believe that this disregards what these passages teach us—that there is a commonality of our history and our identities that is grounded in our breaking of the traditional procreative, sexual, and gender roles.

How does this treatment by an often well-meaning gay and lesbian people affect me? In a very similar way to how the marginalization of gay and lesbian people in the general community affects me as a lesbian. *This treatment separates me from a portion of a shared history, which is often appropriated by gay and lesbian people to the exclusion of transgendered people.* When a person such as Billy Tipton has died and been discovered to have lived life as a member of the sex opposite that of her or his anatomical sex, we are often told that the person was gay or lesbian by most gay and lesbian historians, even though no evidence suggests that the person ever identified as anything other than her or his public gender. Were such people closeted, or transgendered? The latter has rarely been presented to us as an option.

The same is true of much of our common history. Transsexual people did not suddenly appear on the scene in the second half of this century because of the availability of sex reassignment surgery. We always have been around, but we were lumped in with other gender deviants, including gay and lesbian people. However, in the distant past, we were often called eunuchs, because many of us were among those eunuchs that we read about in the ancient texts. In addition, ancient people lumped gay men in with us and called them eunuchs too.

A growing number of gay and lesbian Christians are correctly embracing the image of the eunuch as a liberative one, although most of them are simultaneously ignoring the fact that it is only by analogy that it applies to them. Many of these same gay and lesbian Christians are embarrassed by, or are otherwise uncomfortable with, transgendered people, and hence try to distance themselves from us, even though it is our commonalty that is the basis of their claim to this scriptural heritage! This results in a form of cultural hogging of tradition, which denies to transgendered people our own history and which marginalizes us.

However, it is not only the gay and lesbian community that ignores this connection or this common heritage. Many transsexuals, whose identity is strongly tied in with their sense of gender, resent the fact that they have been mistaken throughout their lives for being gay or lesbian, which challenges their own sense of gender identity. This results in anger directed toward those for whom they are mistaken. But this anger masks the fact that there are some fundamental connections between these otherwise different groups of people, and that even these cases of "mistaken identity" serve to bind us together as a group, albeit one defined by others.

As a result of this anger and our own internalized transphobia, as well as a mistaken tendency to view eunuchs solely as involuntarily castrated men, several of my transsexual sisters with whom I've talked have gotten furious with my identifying myself with the eunuchs. "I'm not just a castrated man; I'm a woman," they shout. They miss the point that I am making, and thereby the liberative message it carries.

This leads to one of my biggest frustrations with the modern gay, lesbian, bisexual, and transgendered community. *We're often too wrapped up in defining ourselves and in defining our own identity, even if that means defining the identity of others.* Too often, the following scenario occurs. A law is passed that intentionally was written to exclude transgendered people, so as not to diminish mainstream political support. Then a cross-dresser is assaulted, fired, or evicted, and the transgendered and gay/lesbian communities jump into a fight over who gets ownership of the victim, while the basher's lawyer tries to dodge around hate crime or nondiscrimination laws saying that the basher was transgender-bashing, which isn't covered! And yet to the basher, this is all nonsense, because to the basher we're all just freaks, and we push all of the basher's buttons about sexuality and gender. Shockingly, the basher instinctively gets something about us that we don't—that we're all bound together in a common oppression, because we're all breaking the same social rules. We're all "queer," in both the best and worst senses of the word.

That's why I find the discussion of procreation and eunuchs so important. The discussion points to the basis of our commonality as sexual minorities. I find it particularly ironic that the most compelling scriptural argument for gay and lesbian affirmation in the Christian scriptures may come from teachings about the transgendered eunuchs, because transgendered people are second-class citizens in the Queer Christian community.

I hope this can be for us a powerful message that brings us together as a gay, lesbian, bisexual, and transgendered community—a community which the ancient scriptures showed was already included in God's love and which would receive a future of acceptance into society as a whole.

NOTES

1. "Oppress" in *The World Book Dictionary*, Volume II. Chicago: Doubleday & Co., 1977, p. 1459.

2. See 2 Sam 3:7 and the annotation to that verse in Bruce M. Metzger and Roland E. Murphy (eds.), *The New Oxford Annotated Bible with the Apocrypha* (New Revised Standard Version). New York: Oxford University Press, 1991.

3. L. William Countryman. *Dirt, Greed & Sex*. Philadelphia: Fortress Press, 1988), pp. 68, 150, 176, 185.

Chapter 4

The Book of Ruth
An Example of Procreative Strategies for Queers

Mona West

Some of the ways the Book of Ruth provides examples of relational and procreative strategies for the lesbian, gay, bisexual, and transgendered community are found in Ruth's love of and devotion to Naomi, which provides a scriptural example of same-sex love. Ruth and Naomi's refusal to accept their fate as childless widows in a society that measured women's worth according to husbands and sons provides the Queer community with an example for refusing to accept our marginalized status as sexual minorities in a heterosexist, patriarchal society. The blessing of the towns-women and the birth of a child to Naomi, Ruth, and Boaz offers a source of blessing for our unions and affirmation of our procreative strategies.

Whether or not we consider ourselves religious, and whether or not we consider the Bible to be the inspired word of God, our reality is that the Bible is used against the Queer community to condemn our lifestyles, exclude us from religious communities, perpetuate violence against us, and deny our basic human rights.

For those of us who choose to enter the debate, we have tradition-ally taken a "defensive" stance toward the ways in which the Bible has been used against our community. We learn a script that includes unpronounceable (not to mention untranslatable) Hebrew and Greek words as well as archaic pagan and Greco-Roman prac-tices of the ancient world. We are faced with nothing less than trying to become biblical scholars in one crash course—"Homo-sexuality and the Bible 101." For others of us, we choose to reject the Bible altogether, claiming, like many feminists, that the texts and the history of their interpretation are "unredeemable."

More recently, Queer folks have taken a different approach to the Bible. Instead of arguing those obscure passages that may or may not say something about same-sex practices in the ancient Near East, we are claiming that Queers actually exist in the Bible and are a significant part of the Judeo-Christian story.

Nancy Wilson, in her book *Our Tribe: Queer Folks, God, Jesus, and the Bible,* identifies quite a cast of us in scripture: eunuchs who appear throughout the Hebrew and Christian scriptures as the ancestors of gay, lesbian, bisexual, and transgendered people; the Ethiopian eunuch of Acts 8—a black, gay man who is the first Gentile convert to Christianity; Lydia, a seller of *purple* in Acts 16:11–15; Mary, Martha, and Lazarus—a nontraditional biblical family, which was Jesus's "family of choice."[1]

Typically, when we think about the existence of gay and lesbian people in the Bible, we think of the stories of Jonathan and David, and Ruth and Naomi. These stories have been variously interpreted as strong friendships, examples of same-sex or bisexual love, oddities in scripture, or relationships that are simple side issues to the much larger roles these characters are supposed to play in the Bible—David, the great king of Israel, and Ruth, the great-grandmother of King David.

I would like to offer a reading of the Book of Ruth that reclaims this story for the Queer community in some powerful ways. The story of Ruth, Naomi, and Boaz is a biblical example of not only same-sex (and possibly sexual) love, but also relational and procreative strategies that are affirming and life-giving for gay, lesbian, bisexual, and transgendered people.

Such a reading is good news to those of us who struggle with the relevance of the Bible in our spiritual journeys. More importantly, the strategies we find in the Book of Ruth are essential to our very survival in a society and culture that invoke narrow definitions of family and procreative privilege in order to exclude us and perpetuate hatred and violence toward our community.

In this chapter-by-chapter analysis of the book of Ruth, the reader is encouraged to follow along in a modern translation of the Bible, such as The New Revised Standard Version, from which I quote,[2] or *Tanakh: A New Translation of the Holy Scriptures.*[3]

"Coming Out" on the Road from Moab to Bethlehem (Ruth 1:1–22)

In a matter of five short verses, a whole family moves from Bethlehem to Moab because of a famine, the father dies, the sons marry Moabite wives, ten years pass, the sons die, and three women are left widowed and childless. The narrative quickly focuses on the situation of the three women: Naomi, the mother-in-law, and her two daughters-in-law, Ruth and Orpah.

There were only two ways a woman could be valued in this society: as an unmarried virgin in her father's household or as a child-producing wife in her husband's household. Naomi is a widow who also becomes childless upon the deaths of her two sons. As childless widows, Naomi, Ruth, and Orpah are women who are worthless and on the margins of ancient Near Eastern society. Naomi recognizes that they have limited options for relationships and for places of "security" in such a society. Naomi admonishes her daughters-in-law not to follow her back to Bethlehem but instead try to find husbands in their homeland of Moab.

We are told that Orpah kisses her mother-in-law good-bye, and that Ruth clings to her. It is at this point in the story that Ruth "comes out" and declares her true feelings for Naomi. In words that have traditionally been repeated in *heterosexual* wedding ceremonies, Ruth speaks to Naomi:

> Do not press me to leave you or to turn back from following you! Where you go, I will go; Where you lodge, I will lodge; your people shall be my people, and your God my God. Where you die, I will die—there will I be buried. May the Lord do thus and so to me, and more as well, if even death parts me from you! (Ruth 1:16)

These words and actions present the closest physical relationship between two women expressed anywhere in the Bible. The Hebrew word that describes Ruth's "clinging" to Naomi is the same word used in Genesis 2:24 to describe the relationship of the man to the woman in marriage. He leaves his father and mother and *clings* to her, and the two become one flesh.

In her words of devotion, Ruth names her relationship to Naomi, using words that depict a relationship that crosses the boundaries of age, nationality, and religion. Ruth chooses against the odds to stay with Naomi—one worthless woman joining herself to another worthless woman. And in her choosing, she refuses to accept the status quo of a society that limits and defines their existence as worthless, empty, and marginal, based on marital status or reproductive ability.

Ruth is our ancestor. She has gone before us and so offers us an example. In her own way, she knew that "silence equals death." After all, Orpah says nothing. According to the story, she kisses Naomi good-bye and promptly disappears. Ruth, however, goes on courageously to name and affirm our relationships in the face of seemingly insurmountable odds. She provides us with an example of self-determination, refusing to accept a marginalized status based on heterosexist, patriarchal definitions of marriage, family, and procreation.

Ruth's words to Naomi in Ruth 1:16 are words for our community. They are pronouncement, blessing, creed, hymn, poem, and declaration, offering paradigms for the ways in which we relate to one another in our comings and goings (*Where you go, I will go*), in our living together (*Where you lodge, I will lodge*), in the communities we create (*your people shall be my people*), and in the ways in which we live and die (*Where you die, I will die—there will I be buried*).

Strategies for Surviving a Hostile Environment (Ruth 2:1–23)

In Chapter 2, Boaz is introduced to the story as a wealthy landowner and a distant relative of Naomi's. After their return to Bethlehem, the women are faced with the day-to-day struggle of providing food for themselves. Israelite law minimally provided for widows and the poor through an ordinance requiring some grain to be left in the fields during harvest for less fortunate to come behind and glean for their food. Ruth knows of this law and decides to go to Boaz's field to glean. Boaz notices her and in true patriarchal fashion asks, "To whom does this young woman belong?" (v. 5). The foreman of the reapers replies, "She belongs to Naomi."

Boaz introduces himself to Ruth, and in stylized, formal language ("Listen my daughter" [v. 8], "Why have I found favor, since I am a foreigner" [v.10]), the two of them acknowledge the relationship that exists between Ruth and Naomi: "All that you have done for your mother-in-law since the death of your husband has been fully told me, and how you left your father and mother and native land and came to a people that you did not know before" (v. 11). These words of Boaz echo Ruth's words of devotion spoken on the road from Moab to Bethlehem in Chapter 1. Not only does Boaz acknowledge their relationship by repeating them, but he invokes God's blessing on their relationship! "May Yahweh reward you for your deeds, and may you have a full reward from Yahweh, the God of Israel, under whose wings you have come for refuge!" (v. 12). In addition to this blessing, Boaz offers extra grain for Ruth and Naomi, and he offers Ruth protection from molestation as she gleans in the fields.

Could it be that Boaz is a gay or bisexual man?* He is characterized in the story as older and unmarried. Could his stylized, formal speech in this chapter be a kind of code that he speaks to Ruth as they come out to each other? He certainly is sympathetic toward Ruth and Naomi. He works out an arrangement with Ruth so that she is able to provide food for herself and Naomi. He also strategizes with Ruth about how to avoid sexual violence in a situation where she is at risk. All of this is done, we are told, at the end of Chapter 2, so that Ruth is able to live with Naomi.

Ruth and Boaz provide the Queer community of today with some strategies for survival in a hostile environment. Contrary to the straw-man stereotype of the wealthy, gay, white man promoted by Christian theocrats, gay, lesbian, bisexual, and transgendered people are often underemployed or unemployed because of internalized homophobia as well as the homophobia of those who would employ us. We may find ourselves homeless, poverty-stricken, or dependent on minimal laws that provide for our well-being. This

---

*I am aware of the complexities of using contemporary words such as *gay* or *bisexual* to describe biblical characters. However, I believe the characterization of Boaz in the story, against the backdrop of ancient Israelite society, indicates something "out of the ordinary" concerning his relationship status—much in the same way that Ruth and Naomi are characterized.

has been especially true for persons living with HIV and AIDS. We are often faced with physical violence in a society that has sexist, misogynist definitions of "real men" and "real women."

The strategy of Ruth and Boaz challenges us to join forces to create communities in which all of us have equal access to goods and services. Like Boaz, those of us with some privilege (those of us who are white, male, able-bodied, educated, and have economic resources) can use those privileges to resist oppressive structures and go above and beyond the law to ensure that those less fortunate in our community are provided for. In many queer communities, we are coming out to one another, acknowledging ways that we can support one another and keep our resources working for the community. Ruth and Boaz remind us that even in the midst of hostile environments, we are able to create communities that affirm our relationships, provide protection, and sustain us.

"We Are Family": Ruth, Boaz, and Me! *(Ruth 3:1–4:11)*

We are told at the end of Chapter 2 that Ruth and Naomi live together under the arrangement Ruth and Boaz have worked out, "until the end of the barley and wheat harvest." At the beginning of Chapter 3, Naomi realizes that a more permanent arrangement must be made, so that it may be well with all of them. (Verse 1 actually reads, "so that it may be well with you.") However, keep in mind that up to this point in the story Ruth has done all the strategizing about how she and Naomi will stay together in a society that refuses to acknowledge their relationship as worthwhile. Naomi's strategy, which follows in Chapter 3, directly involves the well-being and security of Ruth but also includes Boaz as an important member of the "family" Naomi is about to create.

In ancient Israel there was a law that required the brother of a dead man to marry his widow and have a child by her to carry on the male lineage of the clan (Deuteronomy 25: 5–10). There was also a law that required a family member, the next of kin, to buy back (redeem) any family property that may have been sold to pay off a debt (Leviticus 25:25–28). There are hints of these laws in the book of Ruth (see 1:12–13; 3:12–13; 4:1–11); however, it is unclear whether they apply in any way to Boaz. There seems to be some ambiguity concerning Boaz's legal responsibilities as well as his blood relationship to Naomi.

The book of Ruth is also filled with terms and language that describe family and kinship. In Ruth 3:2, Naomi identifies Boaz as a "kinsman." Earlier, Boaz was identified as a "kinsman" of Naomi's on her husband's side, a member of the "tribe" or "clan" of Naomi's deceased husband (2:1). In Ruth 2:20, Naomi identified Boaz as a "nearest kin."

All of these words and laws provide for some interesting narrative possibilities concerning the familial relationship that exists between Ruth, Boaz, and Naomi. Naomi works within these ambiguities to create a situation in which she, Boaz, and Ruth can form their own family to provide security and well-being.

In Ruth 3:1–5, Naomi gives Ruth instructions on how to approach Boaz at night on the threshing floor. These instructions, along with the sexual overtones of the actual encounter between Ruth and Boaz on the threshing floor point to the possibility of Ruth and/or Boaz being bisexual. In verse 9, Ruth proposes marriage to Boaz by invoking the redeemer law of Leviticus 25. In verses 10 and 11, Boaz agrees to marry Ruth, while still acknowledging Ruth's relationship to Naomi: "This instance of your loyalty [to Naomi] is better than the first [returning from Moab with Naomi— see 2:11]."

All of these actions indicate Naomi, Ruth, and Boaz's decision to create their own family and define their own understanding of kinship and responsibility to one another within the context of the inheritance and kinship laws of ancient Israel. These actions parallel the ways in which gay, lesbian, bisexual, and transgendered people of today create families. For example, a bisexual man and two lesbians live together with their biological child; a female-to-male transsexual marries a heterosexual woman; a gay man and a heterosexual woman choose to marry and create family for themselves[4]; a lesbian marries a bisexual man from Mexico in order for him to become a legal immigrant to the United States; three gay men live together as lovers and family while active in the Queer community of San Francisco. The examples could go on and on.

Ruth, Boaz, and Naomi provide our community with an ancient example of the ways in which we have been creating our families through our history as gay, lesbian, bisexual, and transgendered people.

When we read on in the story, we find that Ruth, Boaz, and Naomi must overcome some barriers in the creation of their family. After Boaz and Ruth decide to marry so that the three of them can be family, Boaz remembers there is a nearer kinsman, more closely related to Naomi, who, by law, is required to act as the redeemer.

Once again, it is ambiguous as to the exact nature of these laws in Deuteronomy 25 and Leviticus 25 as they apply to Ruth and Naomi's situation. Within this ambiguity, Boaz manipulates the legal situation so that the nearer kinsman abandons his claim to redeem Naomi and her land. The scene at the city gate (Ruth 4:1–11) shows Boaz at his best in the story. He "sets up" the nearer kinsman by giving just enough information about Naomi and this mysterious land she owns. As the nearer kinsman agrees to redeem the land, Boaz interjects, "Oh by the way, there is this Moabitess named Ruth who is with Naomi—she is also part of the deal. . . . " (Ruth 4:3–5). Out of greed and selfishness (and maybe some ancient Near Eastern homophobia!), the nearer kinsman passes on the option to be family for Naomi and Ruth (v. 6).

As we shall see in the remainder of Chapter 4, Boaz's strategy for overcoming these barriers of inheritance and redemption laws worked. He and Ruth are able to marry, and the family of Ruth, Naomi, and Boaz is recognized by the whole town.

Certainly there are ways that we in the Queer community manipulate laws to overcome barriers that deny the legality of our relationships. We also work the system to make our relationships more permanent and "secure."

We do this through domestic partnerships, which allow us such benefits as health insurance, accident and life insurance, housing and visitation rights, and the use of recreational facilities. We take each other's last names, buy homes together, make wills, give durable power of attorney for health care and finances—all in the face of an ambiguous legal system that discriminates against us.[5] Ruth, Naomi, and Boaz probably would be proud of the ways in which we continue to follow their strategies for creating family and having our relationships recognized.

Blessing Our Unions and Affirming Our Procreative Strategies (Ruth 4:13–22)

In Ruth 4:13, we are told that Ruth and Boaz have a son. The townswomen of Bethlehem have some interesting things to say in response to this birth. They bless the birth and designate the child as "redeemer" ("next of kin," the same word used in Leviticus 25). They claim the child shall be a "restorer of life" for Naomi. They acknowledge Ruth's love for Naomi (this is the only time the word *love* is used in the entire story), and they make the outrageous statement that Ruth is more to Naomi than seven sons! (Remember how important sons were in Chapter 1?) To top all of this off, Naomi breast-feeds* the child, and the townswomen name the child Obed, saying, "A son has been born to Naomi."

In their words and actions the townswomen acknowledge the procreative strategy of Ruth and Boaz that produced a son for Naomi. Their blessing redefines procreation as life-giving. Naomi is not the biological mother of Obed, yet the townswomen realize Ruth's relationship to Naomi has been life-giving—literally in the birth of a son, and spiritually and emotionally in the love of Ruth who, once a worthless widow, is worth more than seven sons to Naomi. The actions of the townswomen in naming the son and Naomi in breast-feeding the child provide examples of the ways in which a whole community is involved in the nourishment and growth of its children.

The gay, lesbian, bisexual, and transgendered community hears the blessing of the townswomen of Bethlehem in our unions. We claim with them that our unions are life-giving, full of love, and worthy. In the words and actions of the townswomen and in the actions of Ruth, Boaz, and Naomi, I am reminded of the procreative strategies our community employs, such as artificial insemination, biological parenting between gay men and lesbians, and adoption.

I am also reminded of the gay male couple of 14 years and the lesbian couple of 12 years who decided to adopt one baby together and have another one through artificial insemination. The four of

---

*It is questionable that the Hebrew text supports such a literal reading. However, the image is evoked for the reader in Naomi's actions and in the context.

them coparent these two beautiful baby girls. I am reminded of the lesbian couple who has been unsuccessful in conceiving a child through artificial insemination and has recently adopted an Asian baby. I am reminded of the naming and blessing of children born to two lesbian couples in my church. The congregation stood facing those children and parents and covenanted with them to participate in their nurture and growth.

In all of these, I hear the townswomen's words of blessing echoing in my heart and ears, "Blessed be Yahweh who has not left you this day without family."

NOTES

1. Wilson, Nancy. *Our Tribe: Queer Folks, God, Jesus, and the Bible.* Harper-SanFrancisco, 1995.

2. *New Revised Standard Version Bible.* National Council of the Churches of Christ, 1989.

3. *Tanakh: A New Translation of the Holy Scriptures.* Philadelphia, New York, and Jerusalem: Jewish Publication Society, 1985.

4. For this story and many others, see Jane Adams Spahr, et al. (Eds.). *Called Out: The Voices and Gifts of Lesbian, Gay, Bisexual, and Transgendered Presbyterians.* Gaithersburg, MD: Chi Rho Press, 1995.

5. For detailed advice concerning legal options for the queer community, see Hayden Curry, Denis Clifford, and Robin Leonard. *A Legal Guide for Lesbian and Gay Couples,* Eighth edition. Berkeley: Nolo Press, 1994.

Chapter 5

Christmas, Sex, Longing, and God
Toward a Spirituality of Desire

Michael Bernard Kelly

We must pay close attention, then, to our liminal experiences, sexual desire, orgasms, loving communion, and spiritual life. We must pay attention to our times of wonder and awe as well as our tastes of quiet, holy presence. We must pay attention to our Christmas mornings.

All my life I have been haunted by longing.

Do you remember Christmas mornings? In our house they used to begin very, very early. After sleeping in fits and starts, one of us children would shake the others awake in the still, predawn darkness, wondering if it was "time" yet. Giggling, with a delicious sense of conspiracy, we would tiptoe breathless and wide-eyed through the slumbering house to peek at the Christmas tree. "Mum! Dad! Father Christmas has been!" The door would be flung open, and we'd be on our knees before all the brightly wrapped marvels, tumbling in anticipation and delight.

If I was lucky, there was at least one special present—one that I couldn't guess at. I'd hold it, shake it, turn it, and wonder what it was. I would unwrap this present slowly, not looking, not wanting to catch a glimpse of a label on the box and guess the secret before the wondrous moment of unveiling. Savoring the edge of possibility, tasting the wonder, I reverently unwrapped this miraculous gift that could be . . . anything! It could be the very thing I longed for, that which I could not name myself, that which I had wanted and waited for, without knowing it, all my life. Could this be it?

There, in that moment, I was on the threshold; I was touching the hem. (Was this how the woman in the Gospel felt when she touched the hem of Jesus' garment, hoping to be made well [Luke 8: 43–48]?)

Eventually, inevitably, the present was unwrapped. Immediately, something wondrous was lost. This was not *It*. And yet . . . there was that moment, that luminous moment when everything was possible. Such a moment! Even today something in me rises to meet it, wide-eyed and, perhaps, even open-hearted.

Why do adults so love Christmastime, so often reflecting that "It's just not the same without children"? I believe the sweetness of this moment lingers. Something in us all is still waiting, still longing, still hoping. Just to be here again on this threshold is delight, as we see shining in the eyes of children our own wonder and hope. Perhaps this year! We are all lost children, waiting on the threshold for the wonder to show itself. We are all haunted by longing.

Do you remember your first orgasm? I remember mine. I didn't really know what it was. I was used to the excitement and pleasure of arousal, but this was completely new and unexpected. I remember very clearly saying to myself that it felt in that moment as if everything I had ever wanted had been given to me. Everything. Not this and that, but the Essence—It. I had tasted that for which I longed. In that brief splinter of time, all was ecstatically complete and fulfilled.

Yet, even as it burst into my life, it was gone. Of course, I soon learned I could taste this delight again and again, and despite the turmoil, chaos, and guilt that came to accompany it, the purity and power of that moment of ecstasy remained, firing my longing and undoing both my own plans and the dictates of a repressed and frightened Church. Again and again I would stand on the threshold and, unlike the Christmas present, this did not disappoint. Here, however fleetingly, I crossed the threshold and tasted the wonder. Yet, like Christmas, it too was gone in the very moment of its sweetest delight.

Do you remember your first taste of spiritual joy? As a boy I had been very religious, loving ritual, prayer, and "holy things." However, when I was about fourteen years old, something new broke into my life. One day when I was spending a lonely lunchtime in the school chapel trying some simple methods of prayer that I had read about, I had a sudden sense of immediate, mirror-like contact with the One to whom I prayed. It was simple, no visions or lights or anything; it was intoxicating, like drinking at a fountain of joy. For several months this continued, especially after Holy Communion when I alternately felt as if I were flying as high as the ceiling or as if I were about to burst from joy. God only knows what my school-mates, bored by the daily liturgy, must have thought as I closed my eyes and drank from this hidden spring.

Again, I was on the threshold, again tasting It; yet It withdrew. Soon the spring dried up, went underground, and my prayer became plain and dry. However, I had known what it was to have my heart on fire, and I would never be satisfied until it consumed me com-pletely.

These three sacred moments—the gift giving of Christmas, sexual awakening, and spiritual awakening—can be called "limi-nal" experiences. *Limen* is the Latin word for "threshold," and it refers in a special way to the threshold of the temple, which is an entrance, a barrier, a meeting place between the sacred and the secular, between the divine and the human, between my deepest self and my ordinary, daily self. In liminal states we taste a deeper level of awareness beyond the rational, analytical, and image-making mind, sometimes even tasting the deepest center of self that opens into the Absolute Mystery, that ground of our being where "God's Spirit with her own Being is effective."[1]

These liminal experiences cannot be controlled by the individual, Church, or society. They take us beyond, and that is the point. They are profoundly free and freeing, shaking up all the structures of the self, unmistakably asserting the sovereign freedom of God in the heart and soul of each person. They come in many ways and with many textures. I have mentioned only three, and in this essay I wish to talk specifically about only two—the spiritual and the sexual.

It is especially in these two areas that society and the Church set out to claim, construct, sanction, and control the liminal experience. This happens primarily through the structures of marriage and offi-cial religious ritual. Some experiences, some pathways into the Mystery become hallowed, celebrated, enshrined, even made man-datory, while others are forbidden, condemned, denied, and even demonized. Some people and their experiences are "in," and other people and their experiences are "out." However, true liminal experiences cannot be legislated. Indeed, in them, a deep freedom and truth are discovered—touchstones to test the preaching and posturing of the institutions themselves, if we have the integrity and the courage.

All the same, it is not simply malice and power that lead society and the Church to try to control and issue caveats about these experiences. That which is tasted in them, whether it comes through prayer, sex, nature, drugs, dance, or ritual is intensely powerful, even overwhelming. Wisdom, prudence, and guidance are essential in the drinking of this water, and a little taste goes a long way. We all know, I suspect, the seductive tendency to seek the thrill of the liminal moment again and again at the expense of "ordinary" life, relationships, and commitments, ultimately forfeiting the true transformation to which the liminal moment points.

First, if we are to be fully human and free, it is essential that we become profoundly open and deeply attentive to our own liminal experiences, especially in our sex and prayer lives. There can be no true spirituality or growth without this. The wisdom of the ages is vital, but we must live our own lives and live from our own deepest center, which is sensed and glimpsed in these moments. We must embrace them, even as we are embraced in them. Better yet, we must embrace not the liminal moment itself nor its context (church, sex, dance, drugs, nature, etc.), but rather we must embrace that which the liminal moment reveals to us, that Mystery, the essence that we taste and to which we surrender, inarticulate, utterly free. We must embrace and drink deeply of the Mystery whenever, wherever, however, and in whomsoever It reveals itself. Laws must not stop us.

Elsewhere I have referred to this as "telling the truth," first to ourselves and then to others.[2] Let us drink deeply, letting the "chips" of social, religious, and personal structures fall where they may in that moment. Can we who are ourselves "on the edge," whose spiritual and sexual experiences are so routinely condemned and denied, have the courage to "drink of the truth" and to proclaim it to others, witnessing to the freedom of the Spirit who will not be articulated, legislated, or controlled, who "blows wherever she wills" (John 3:8)? Here is a truly prophetic, revolutionary, and human vocation!

What then of the wisdom and prudence of which I spoke earlier? And what of the inevitable, all too immediate moment when the tasting, embracing, and showing are gone, and we either tumble deliciously in its wake like dolphins behind a ship or feel the chaos and emptiness it has stirred up in our stagnant pond of a life?

This withdrawing, this hide-and-seek, is the other essential quality of the liminal experience. It must be faced. All too often we who are excluded from so much that society and Church hold dear cling tenaciously to the thrill of the moment, seeking it over and over again, compulsively, even desperately, "like vultures fighting over a corpse," as a gay friend put it recently. We must allow the withdrawing. We must let go.

When Heidegger says, "That which itself shows itself and at the same time withdraws is the essential trait of what we call the Mystery,"* he is expressing a truth that all of us know at a deep, soul level. We also know it in our bodies. Perhaps the experience of orgasm is the clearest example of this for most of us. In that very moment of ecstasy, in that tasting, that bliss, that knowing, that briefest communion with that which cannot be named, as we are thrown over the peak of consciousness, at the burning "white-hot tip of sexuality"[3] as It shows itself, It withdraws. We are left astonished, filled, and shattered by sex, but we are left.

What is going on here? Is God playing games with us? Are we being enticed, teased, and abandoned? It is relevant to state that these precise questions are also faced in the spiritual life of prayer, as the One who set our hearts on fire seems to abandon us, and we are "left on the streets," "beaten," "wounded," and "stripped" like the bride in the Song of Songs (5:7). This is a serious question, and in our longing we ask it from the depths of our heart.

Could it be that this showing and withdrawing actually reveals to us something of the nature of the Mystery, itself; something of our own nature, and something of the nature of human transformation?

---

*Heidegger, Martin. *Discourse on Thinking*. A translation of his *Gelassenheit* by John M. Anderson and E. Hans Freund. New York: Harper & Row, 1966, p. 55. I am indebted to Fr. John Dunne, C.S.C., for his reflections on the nature of human longing and especially for his statement from Heidegger, and also for Dunne's concept of "Shapes of Longing." My interpretation and use of these concepts in this essay are, however, my own.

Could it be essential to the spiritual journey? In the Book of Exodus, Moses, after receiving the Law, asks to see God's face. God tells Moses to hide in the cleft of a rock and as he passes, God will shield him with his hand, and Moses can look out and see God's back (Exodus 33:18–23). It would be death to see God face-to-face, not in the sense of being punished, but because the encounter would be overwhelming and unbearable. It would shatter the container of the human.

To encounter the Mystery, the Unnameable One, who is God, is to go beyond words, concepts, images and doctrines, and to stand naked, utterly vulnerable in the embrace of the ineffable essence of That Which Is, encountering It in ourselves, as ourselves, as all. This is that which "no eye has seen, no ear has heard, nor has it entered into the mind of humans to conceive" (I Corinthians 2:9). This encounter can only be borne in the briefest of touches; a full revelation of the Mystery is literally unthinkable, impossible for human life as we now live it. Even our fleeting glimpses baffle and stun us.

In the immediate withdrawing of the Mystery, even as it embraces us, as it licks our lips, we see its nature as utterly "more," ultimately "beyond," and transcending all, just as in its showing we see its immanence, for it is closer to us than we are to ourselves, intimate and immediate in the depths of our humanness.

In our truly liminal experiences, in the depths of prayer and in the depths of sex, I believe we do indeed encounter this Absolute Mystery, showing and withdrawing, embracing and emptying, and we long for it with all our hearts and souls! "My body pines for you, like a dry weary land without water," cries the Psalmist (Psalms 63:1), and the mystic and the lover in us cry out with him. We know the yearning of those who "are willing to make shipwrecks of themselves to gain the one they love."[4] It is the withdrawing of the Mystery that kindles and rekindles this longing.*

Here, then, is the second gift of the withdrawing—that it seduces us onto the spiritual journey, which is the human quest for maturity,

---

*Dunne, J.S., loc cit. This "showing and withdrawing" of the Mystery, and the "emptying and embracing" reflect the two great movements of the Christian spiritual life: the Apophatic (negative) Way and the Cataphatic (affirmative) Way.

union, and transformation. In every era and in every part of life, there is a tendency for us to focus on experiences, ecstatic thrills, the tastes and touches already discussed. This tendency is especially marked in sexuality and spirituality, where the tastes are so intoxicating, fleeting, and profound. These tastes are essential; they are seeds, glimpses of that fullness to which we are called. However, they are not the journey, itself; not transformation; not mystical union; and not enlightenment. They set us on the road; perhaps they are even glimpses of the destination, but we have not yet arrived. Indeed we have hardly set out! If we become addicted to simply seeking more and more experiences, whether sexual or spiritual, we never will arrive. We all know this tendency in sexuality, but the seduction in spirituality can be more subtle, more compelling, and more soul destroying.

So what is happening? Some element of this addiction is probably inevitable in our yearning and longing for the taste of ecstasy. However it comes, it is so delicious, and overwhelming—of course we seek it again and again!

"You shed your fragrance about me; I drew breath and now I gasp for your sweet perfume. I tasted you and now I hunger and thirst for you. You touched me and I am inflamed with love of your peace," says Saint Augustine,[5] and in our different ways we know what he means. However, we must allow the withdrawing to take place. It is the withdrawing that will draw us toward the transformation to the abiding fulfillment of that which we taste so briefly in our ecstasies. How does this happen?

When we taste the Mystery, we long to drink deeply of it, to take it into ourselves, to be possessed by it, to surrender to it, to become it in an abiding way, "forever and ever." I think of our images of sexual hunger and thirst, not just our desire to "do it" with a particular person, but to "drink them in," "gobble them up," nibble, lick, suck, and swallow—all the metaphors of eating and delights of sex. This is mirrored very powerfully in the images of spiritual communion, where we eat and drink "the body and blood of the Lord," our very bodies merging and becoming transformed into the One who is the beloved of our souls.

This is the heart of our yearning—to become that which we taste and hunger for, not briefly but fully, totally, and permanently, being utterly transformed into that which we desire so deeply, which is union and ecstasy—the "Lover with his beloved / transforming the beloved in her Lover,"[6] the seeker transformed into that which she seeks.

This truly is to die to ourselves, to lose our life so as to find it (Luke 9:24), to enter into the mystery of death and resurrection. This is what we hunger and thirst for in our bodies, in our sexuality no less than in our spirituality, and this is what we taste in both. All that is deeply and authentically human is a pathway into this transformation, but sexuality and spirituality draw us most profoundly, most ecstatically. I think of Jesus speaking to the woman at the well (John 4:5–42), seducing her into her spiritual journey with the promise of a spring of living water that would never run dry. We taste this spring, and we thirst for the day when rivers of this living water will rise within us, flow out of our "bellies," and well up to eternal life, eternal union, and eternal love (John 7:38).*

The Mystery that shows Itself must withdraw. It must seduce us. It must play a game of "now, not yet" with us, enticing us, leading us on and on, inflaming our longing at deeper and deeper levels, teaching us that the taste of this "water" is not enough, allowing us to find both bliss and bitterness in the tasting (especially when we become "hooked"). It must teach us to follow the withdrawal, to let go and go deeper, learning the lessons of how to become in the abiding, ordinary, everyday reality of our lives—that which we taste and for which we thirst. Nothing less will satisfy our hunger, fulfill our longing, or transform our humanity into the divinity we seek.

How does this look in practice, in people's actual lives? It is important to say that there are as many answers to this question as there are people to ask it. The human journey of transformation, although it has universal qualities, is profoundly personal and particular and will look very different to each of us as we experience growth and purification in ways we least expect but most need.[7]

---

*There are those who would applaud these words as applied to "holy longing" and "spiritual desires" of the soul, but would wish to accord sexual yearning a lower place. I refer them to the Mystery of the Incarnation. There is one hunger, one thirst, one longing, one love moving in the depths of all that we are. We feel this most powerfully, most physically in our longing for sexual intimacy and ecstasy.

Those of us marginalized by mainstream society, both secular and religious, because of our sexuality need to remember this, as does anyone who seeks to guide us. The ways we experience and embody our deepest longings often look very different from the ways sanctioned by a heterosexist culture, and consequently our path of transformation will look very different. In us the free, uncontrolled Spirit of God offers a gift to humanity, freeing others to embrace this journey so particular, yet so universal. We must dare to be different; we must risk becoming our true selves.

What then are the universal qualities of the transforming journey? They are many, and there are many books written about them in all religions. However, the "bottom line," I believe, is the fact that in the end we are all longing for the same thing. In our spiritual practices, in our sexual desire, in the lives and relationships we build, through all the fetishes, dreams, and different "shapes" our longing has taken over the years—when all these have run their course, worn out, or faded away—we will find that we are all longing for communion with the Other and for self-transcendence, in and through that communion. We long for communion, transcendence, intimacy, and ecstasy.

From the first orgasm, and in every orgasm since, I have sought that ecstatic moment, and its allure still colors so much of my life. I seek out its possibility, feel its approach, surrender to it, and allow the rigid sense of self to melt deliciously as it rises within me, letting myself be caught up in the juicy passion that draws me toward it. There is an aloneness in this, as I close my eyes and go deeply into my experience of pleasure and let the ecstatic flow become all that I am. There is a deep solitude in the drinking of this water.

However, I also long to share this ecstatic vulnerability with another person, and that which I seek to drink in ecstasy I am drawn to in and through other persons. Put simply, I long to have sex with another person, however intense solitary sexual pleasure may be. At a conference on AIDS, I once tried to persuade a church group that we needed to reassess the potential goodness and grace in all kinds of sexual relating, including "recreational sex." An agitated woman finally snapped at me, "Well, why can't you just masturbate!" I snapped back, "I do, don't you?" My real answer, however, would be that it simply is not the same. There is another whole dimension of life—and of ecstasy itself—present in my relating with another, or other persons, whether it be in a casual encounter or in a lifelong relationship. This other dimension is communion and intimacy.

As one matures, this desire for communion deepens, and the ecstatic moment seems somewhat incomplete, even empty, without this growing, broadening communion with another, with the other in others, in all the dimensions of one's life and personality. At the same time, it must be kept in mind that without the allure and ecstatic possibility of self-transcendence in and through our relating, communion can all too easily become complacent and tasteless (and we go out looking!).

So, we long for communion and transcendence. We long for them and sometimes experience them as separate and sometimes as intimately interwoven. At a deep level, however, they are two faces of the same Mystery: Love. It is clear that those we call "lovers" seek the truth of this. I see it, too, quite graphically in the desire to climax with the person with whom I am having sex. We also see it in the Christian spiritual teaching that the saintly hermit and the saintly activist are both, at depth, ecstatically transcending self and simultaneously in communion with God and with all beings—solitude and union; communion and transcendence; intimacy and ecstasy; Love.

This longing for communion and transcendence is the essence of spirituality; it is what I seek when I pray, what I try to live out in service, what I call true holiness when it matures in a human being. This is the same mystery that I long for in sex, in the daily reality of my life, in my choices, relationships, and dreams. It is not esoteric and exotic, but ordinary and human, like true spirituality. It is this ordinariness, this humanness, this embodiedness that opens onto divinity. We will find it at home—in our cells, in our sweat.

This opening onto divinity is the truth of all that is genuinely human and cannot be restricted by the dictates of Church and society. Often, it will happen most profoundly in people and in situations outside the approved norms, where people are on the edge, seeking to follow their hearts, having only their thirst for their guide. Saints, lovers, artists, and mystics have never been fit for polite society. They drink from the same well, perhaps in different ways and at different depths, but it is the same thirst and the same water. Little wonder, then, that their passionate language of love so often sounds the same!

However, mystics and lovers also know, if they are honest, that the Mystery, which shows itself in intimacy and ecstasy, also withdraws. We have looked at one dimension of this withdrawing. Is there another?

We long for communion and self-transcendence. In our sex and in our prayer we taste this. Sometimes this ecstatic, intimate experience is especially deep and comes through a particular person or in a particular context. We feel a profound allurement. Here is the chance to drink deeply and abidingly of this water, to be possessed by and to possess the Mystery, to be transformed, become what we taste, to have all our dreams come true! We make life choices on the basis of this liminal experience of allurement and possibility. We form relationships, join communities, serve the poor, get married, learn Tantric sex, choose celibacy, take up a spiritual practice, or move to the beach. All of these are shapes our longing takes at certain moments, and sometimes throughout many years, and we embrace them hoping to drink deeply and to become what we taste in and through a particular person, practice, or path. We celebrate and send out invitations!

Sooner or later, however, the camellias turn brown, the honeymoon ends, and we ask ourselves, "Who is this at the breakfast table?" My God, what have I done? Sooner or later the Mystery withdraws. What now?

The first thing to say, again, is that the Mystery must withdraw. However holy or sexy this person, practice, or path may be, the Divine Mystery lies both in and beyond him, her, or it. We cannot fulfill one another's deepest longings. In this sense, I am not God. I am not the beloved of another's soul, for I, too, am seeking that beloved. When I "fall in love," part of what is happening is that I am projecting my own longing for union with the Mystery onto another person. The poet Rilke says that lovers are close to the Mystery: "It opens up to them behind each other." However, they are "blocking each other's view," and "neither one can get past."[8] Someday we obscurely realize this, and we say things like, "You're not the man I married!" and in a certain sense that's right.

However, this realization, this withdrawing of the Mystery teaches us to do what we can do—to nurture, support, love, and encourage one another on our own spiritual journey, recognizing, too, that in our lovemaking we do indeed encounter the depths of one another, those depths that go beyond the individual and into absolute communion. Then we can, perhaps, join hands and go forward side by side rather than face to face.

Even in this, however, we must face the fact that the person or people we love will one day die, and yet our longing will go on and on beyond them and into death itself. This is also true of spiritual paths, practices, and teachings. They are all fingers pointing to the moon, as Zen has it. Even Jesus said that he was the "gate" (John 10:9) and "the way" (John 14:6). The finger, the gate, and the way are not the destination! We must follow the direction of the finger, go through the gate, walk the way, trusting more and more, and leaving behind all that is familiar and safe. We must embrace the Mystery.

The shapes of my longing, the shapes the Mystery seems to take in my life must play their part, but they must also fail. A gracious "letting go" is what we are called to, but this process is usually deeply painful, even shattering, and can feel as if it is destroying the soul. All that we cling to—all of our old ambitions, values, and loves—will be stripped away, sometimes gradually, sometimes violently. There is nowhere to hide, except in illusion. If we can be open enough, if we can wait, if we can slowly accept the gift of trust in the midst of darkness and desolation, we will come to sense in our loneliness and emptiness a deeper, silent, "dark" embrace of the Mystery. In the emptying is the embrace.

This can only happen for me in the depths of my true self, and there is profound solitude in this. The person or path "out there" may have helped me "come home" to my deep self, but as I do, I must release him, her, or it to be free to enter the silence of this dark embrace. Furthermore, it is in the ending of the honeymoon phase of relationships, lovemaking, spiritual life, and sex that we glimpse what it might actually mean to become that which we taste. It is communion and self-transcendence that we seek. Sooner or later we must learn what it means to live this out every day, in the ordinary, mundane, unexciting, "nonliminal" reality of life. We must learn what it means to transcend self again and again, not just in ecstasy but in taking out the garbage, in the boredom and interior anguish of prayer, in the stink of the poor, or of a dying lover whom we once embraced so passionately because he or she seemed to us like heaven itself. We must learn the endless concern, generosity, sensitivity, and forgiveness that living a life of communion with the Other demands. This is practical, down-to-earth, simple, and incredibly demanding. This is the other side of losing one's life so as to save it, of death and resurrection, of becoming a lover. A transformed human being lives a real life of days, hours, and minutes; of cleaning, cooking, and recreation; of listening, speaking, laughing, and crying.

There is a Buddhist saying, "After enlightenment—the laundry!" One might also say, "Before, during, and on the way to enlightenment—the laundry!" We are not playing games here; we are not seeking just liminal thrills for all their beauty and power. The Mystery must withdraw into the ordinariness of the everyday, for that is the place of learning and of transformation.

In the midst of this hard work of becoming, however, there will still be tastes and glimpses of that which we seek. These refresh, renew, and encourage us, and they are vital. As the years pass, however, these will have different, deepening textures, perhaps quieter, perhaps more free, sometimes more searing and overwhelming. Gradually the intimacy and the ecstasy will become one. Gradually, too, we will begin to sense a quiet, abiding embrace in the foundation of our soul.

In the maturity of the spiritual life, the sexual life, the human life, there is a peace and a surrender that is a still, abiding passion which runs gentle and deep. The fireworks are few; they accompanied the momentary collapse of the structures of self that allowed earlier tastes of the Mystery. Now these structures are simpler, softer, more saturated with the presence of the Divine. One thinks of the classic image of the old couple (at least as often gay or lesbian as straight) whose intimacy flows quietly, needing few words or thrilling experiences. They abide in and with each other, loved and known, knowing and loving. I think, too, of the wise old Indian teacher to whom Ram Dass offered LSD to see what would happen. The teacher took it, smiled, and just went on sitting, meditating in unitive peace. He was already there.*

Old age, of course, is not essential in spiritual growth.** In Randy Shilts' book, *And the Band Played On,* he tells the story of Gary Walsh, a gay man in San Francisco who went through the different phases of "AIDS is a spiritual gift" and "AIDS is an ugly curse" to finally reach a simple, deep tranquility before he died. On the day he died a friend told him of the effect he was having on others, that people were coming away from conversations with him "like pilgrims leaving a holy shrine."

> Gary smiled his mischievous grin and interrupted her. "I got it, I finally got it," he said. "I am love and light and I transform people by just being who I am." Gary recited the words carefully, like a schoolchild who had struggled hard to master a difficult lesson.[9]

Many of us have seen such simple, human holiness firsthand in our friends and lovers. Many of us are growing toward it right now. This holy, human maturity is based on our readiness to respond to the deepest challenges of learning, trusting, surrendering, loving, becoming open not only to the embrace but also to the painful emptying, to the showing and the withdrawing, allowing the shapes of longing to fail and fall away, leaving only "love—longing."[10] We become that which we taste.

We must pay close attention, then, to our liminal experiences: sexual desire, orgasms, loving communion, and spiritual life. We must pay attention to our times of wonder and awe, as well as to our tastes of quiet, holy presence. We must pay attention to our Christmas mornings. Equally, we must be open to our emptying and to the "school of love"*** that is everyday life. Most of all, we must listen

---

*In the 1960s, Ram Dass, with Timothy Leary, was one of the early experimenters with LSD. Disillusioned with the transitory nature of the experience it offered, he traveled to India in search of more abiding transformation. See Ram Dass. *Be Here Now*. New Mexico: Hanuman Foundation, 1971.

**That remarkable contemplative, St. Therese of Lisieux, who died of Tuberculosis in 1897 at the age of 24, is proof enough of this.

***Jones, A. *Soulmaking*. London: SCM Press, 1985, p. 1. This is an ancient term referring to the discipline of monastic life.

to our longing, not simply our desire for this or that person, but to the longing that rises from the center of our hearts and that leads us on and on through the years, into and beyond our loves, as familiar and profound as breathing. In the embracing and the emptying, this center will become our place of stillness and truth. In the moment of death, it is through this center that our longing will pass, opening us to the "first Alleluia! of [our] eternity"[11] and to the eternal dance of desire with the Absolute Mystery of Love in whom we will be transformed from Glory to Glory!*

It is for this that we were born; it is this that we taste; it is to this that we are destined—lesbian, gay, bisexual, transgender, and straight. It is our birthright.

> "Unnameable God, my essence;
> my origin, my lifeblood, my home."[12]

And it all begins in the honest, earthy, human desire for love, sex, communion, and self-transcendence. It all begins in that moment just before a small child opens the much-longed-for Christmas present.

All my life I have been haunted by longing.

NOTES

1. Meister Eckhart quoted in Fox, M. *Original Blessing*. New Mexico: Bear and Co., 1983, p. 132.

2. See my videocourse titled "The Erotic Contemplative: The Spiritual Journey of the Gay/Lesbian Christian." Erospirit Research Institute: Oakland, CA, 1994, Volume 1.

3. Browning, F. *The Culture of Desire*. New York: Crown Publishers Inc., 1993, p. 88.

4. Burrows, R. *Ascent to Love*. London: Darton, Longman and Todd, 1987, p. 115.

5. Saint Augustine. *Confessions*. Translated by R.S. Pine-Coffin. Middlesex: Penguin Classics, 1961, p. 232 (Book X, Chapter 27).

---

*St. Gregory of Nyssa saw the life of heaven as an eternal progression into God as our desire is constantly kindled, fulfilled, and rekindled at deeper levels. See for example his *Life of Moses*. Quoted and translated by H. Musurillo in his *From Glory to Glory: Texts from Gregory of Nyssa*. London: John Murray, 1962, pp. 142–148.

6. St. John of the Cross. *The Dark Night.* st.5. Translated by K. Kavanaugh, O.C.D. and Otilio Rodriguez, O.C.D. Washington, DC: ICS Publications, 1973, p. 296.

7. Burrows. op. cit., pp. 108–109. Burrows shows how the "Dark Night" can look very different according to people's varying needs and personalities.

8. Rilke, R.M. *Duino Elegies.* Translated by D. Young. New York: Norton and Co.,1978, p. 73 (Eighth Elegy).

9. Shilts, R. *And the Band Played On.* New York: St. Martin's Press, 1987, p. 425.

10. Julian of Norwich. *Showings.* Translated by Edmund Colledge and James Walsh. New York: Paulist Press, 1978, p. 318.

11. From the saying of Pedro Arrupe, S.J., regarding death. Quoted by John J. McNeil in his lecture, "Drinking from Our Own Wells," September 26, 1991. Berkeley, CA.

12. Psalm 19:14. Translated by Stephen Mitchell. in *The Enlightened Heart.* New York: Harper & Row, 1989, p. 7.

SECTION II.
FAMILIES OF CHOICE

Having deconstructed the myth that only one woman and one man, joined under the auspices of government, along with their progeny, can constitute a family, we are left to examine a variety of kin connections that have long been ignored or discounted. Some of these are created out of love, some out of choice, and some are merely the result of the genetic lottery.

Chapter 6

The Power to Choose
We're Here, We're Queer, and We Want to Get Hitched

Amy Adams Squire Strongheart

The Holy Spirit had revealed to me, mostly through the conscientious instruction of my free-thinking Protestant parents, that I could not blame the Bible, the preacher, the teacher, or even my parents, themselves, for my decisions. And I realized at that monumental juncture in my life that I could not surrender my personal power to any moral agent or authority. Ultimately, whether I decided to live the lie of "heterosexual impersonation" or to live with integrity in a same-sex union, despite the social condemnation that would surely result, I would be accountable for that decision and responsible for the consequences of it.

In July 1991, on a lovely, temperate day (a rarity in hot, humid St. Louis), I was married in an Episcopal church to Alexah Strongheart. She is the golden-haired, blue-eyed Norse Goddess whose happy task is to keep me from taking myself too seriously. Our wedding invitation read as follows:

This day I will marry my friend,
the one I laugh with, live for, love.
Amy Adams Squire *and* **Carrie Bernice Clement**
invite you to witness the blessing of their relationship
as they become
Amy Adams Squire Strongheart
and
Carrie Alexah Strongheart

It is absolutely astounding how many uninformed Heterosexuals think that all Lesbians, Gays, and Bisexuals[1] do is engage in gratuitous sex without bothering to court or commit.

"Fundies,"[2] those arbiters of "moral correctness" and the most formidable adversaries of the Lavender[3] civil and human rights movement, insist that God mandated marriage and that it should be compulsory. Even so, they are the first to call a press conference denouncing same-sex couples the right to marry. Go figure.

In the pages that follow, I assert from personal conviction and experience that we are created by God with the capacity for love (and lots of it), and we are therefore entitled to pledge ourselves to each other as we see fit. I also affirm our right and ability to draw from those traditions with which we are familiar and comfortable.

The underlying supposition of this essay is that although Lavender people do not yet have all the same *privileges,* such as legalized marriage, that the dominant heteropatriarchal cultures of this planet enjoy, we do have *power*—personal power. Personal power is the ability to choose who we are and how to live our lives as who we are, rather than allowing someone else to define through tyranny our identity or the parameters of our existence for us. In some cultures, namely Western ones, it is easier and safer to access that personal power. Nonetheless, that power is available to all of us, and it is our God-given right to exercise it.

One of the ways I learned this was through my own journey through the matrimonial maze. I recall that during the year of premarital counseling that Alexah and I received, one of the first things I had to address was my own residual, internalized fear of being a Lesbian. Remarkably, after being out of the closet for nearly a decade, I was caught unawares by the demon of homophobia,[4] which apparently had not been entirely exorcised from my consciousness.

The interpretations imposed on the "texts of terror,"[5] which most Gays, religious and nonreligious, have heard pontificated *ad nauseam,* threatened to turn my dream of wedded bliss into a nightmare. Could this be some kind of cruel joke, I wondered, where, upon dying, my soul would ascend to the throne of judgment and receive the penalty of perdition for failing to accept compulsory heterosexuality?

What to do? I recalled past experiences in which every time I had sought direction about who I was and how God wanted me to live in the world, I was gently led further down the path of self-acceptance and self-affirmation. The Holy Spirit had revealed to me, mostly through the conscientious instruction of my free-thinking Protestant parents, that I could not blame the Bible, the preacher, the teacher, or even my parents, themselves, for my decisions. And I realized at that monumental juncture in my life that I could not surrender my personal power to any moral agent or authority. Ultimately, whether I decided to live the lie of "heterosexual impersonation" or to live with integrity in a same-sex union, despite the social condemnation that would surely result, I would be accountable for that decision and responsible for the consequences of it.

But I still harbored skepticism about the grace I had been shown. What if those intransigent old Fundies were right? What if I and my lovely Bisexual bride-to-be really were an ABOMINATION to God?

This unexpected bout of self-deprecation sent me straight (no pun intended) to the priest. "What if I'm not really a Lesbian," I wailed. "What if I *chose* to be this way?"

The priest looked at me incredulously. Then composing herself, she looked me right in my terrified and tearful eyes and said, "Well, what if you did? What difference does it make?"

Hello? Was it possible that the nature versus nurture nonsense about sexual orientation was irrelevant to Divine determination of human absolute value? In the quest for Lavender liberation, to be treated as equals to Heterosexuals, we have made much of the argument that we have no latitude in matters concerning to whom we are spiritually, emotionally, psychologically, and sexually attracted. We often pose the question in reverse to prove our point: Do Heterosexuals choose to be Heterosexual?

Although there is much merit in this line of reasoning, it has failed us in that such thinking does not *empower* us. It forces us to be *victims* of our nature. Would we ever choose to be Lesbian, Gay, or Bisexual because these are holy, joyous, and special natures? Oh, no. We insist that biology has made the decision for us, and we would magically be transformed into Heterosexuals if only we could. God knows we wouldn't purposely identify as members of one of the most despised and abused minorities in the world. Poor us.

I once spoke to a group of about 60 senior citizens, one of whom asked me if I could be reborn as a Straight person, would I? My answer was, "No." I'm very comfortable being a Lesbian. In addition, I have learned so much about so many things like love, decency, tolerance, family, gender, intimacy, and personal responsibility—all lessons that I might not have learned had I not incarnated as a Lesbian. And I do believe I had a vote in my incarnation.

I take a rather metaphysical approach to my Lesbianism. Jesus said, "You judge according to the flesh,"[6] and we do. We assess one another according to race, ethnicity, religion, class, sex, sexual orientation, weight, height, personality, and physical and mental ability. These are all purely incidental characteristics although not irrelevant. There is a part of each of us that is as perfect, consistent, and timeless as the loving Divine Mind from which it was conceived. But we are each individual and unique expressions of that magnificent divinity, and to discount any part of that incarnation is to deny the will of God, which is what, in my estimation, accounts for so much of the fear, resentment, and discord in the world.

This is, then, the greatest lesson I have learned, which is that *God loves me because of who I am and not in spite of who I am.*

We have a *moral obligation* to be who we are as well as to choose who we will be and to carve out our niche in this world accordingly. Because we *are* the will of God, we are therefore obliged to promote same-sex marriage as a holy, decent, and legitimate estate worthy of affirmation.

Before launching into a grand polemic about how we might accomplish this, I would first like to suggest that marriage is a purely social construct. My suspicions about the transience of marriage were aroused by Matthew 22:23–33, in which Jesus fields a question thrown at him by one of the Marcia Clarks of his day. The prosecutor cleverly inquires of the rabbi which of a man's seven wives would be with him in the afterlife.

First of all, Jesus manages to point out in that charming, understated way of his (and I paraphrase liberally here) that in their convoluted mental masturbation, the Sadducees had missed the point entirely. Next he says, "In the resurrection they neither marry nor are given in marriage, but are like angels in heaven." I take that to mean that marriage is an arrangement suitable for our temporal life here on earth. Perhaps it is to help us express the divine love of heaven that is the part of our deepest nature. So why not derive maximum benefit from it?

To procure such benefit, however, we first have to decide what marriage is. Let me state right up front that *it is each individual's right to decide for herself or himself what marriage is,* and there are innumerable legal, social, religious, cultural, and individual definitions of marriage. Here's mine: *A marriage is a covenant of love between two consenting adults[7] who must be as committed to the covenant as they are to each other, and they must live out their covenant on a daily basis.*

I do not believe that marriage can be coerced; it cannot exist between two children or between an adult and a child, and it cannot exist between more than two persons. However, as a caveat, I would say that the love upon which the marriage covenant is based ought to bring out the best not only in the partners but also in the community in which they reside. In this respect, then, a marriage is not limited to just two persons because the fruits of that love bless all who receive them.

Alexah and I have discovered that one of the reasons our marriage has endured is that we have developed a loyalty, not just to each other, but to the covenant of marriage, itself. We believe our marriage to be a *sacred calling*. In addition, we have found that the marriage did not begin, nor did it end, with the recitation of the vows (see p. 92). To fulfill our calling as a couple in covenant, we must practice our pledge as best we can each day. Since life is dynamic and not static, each day is different, and we must adapt our promises to the flow of our life together.[8]

So how do Lavender people honor that holy vocation one day at a time? We need to develop a model of matrimony that works for us.

I am not of the opinion that marriage must be mandatory for everyone—especially not the Heterosexual model of marriage. Again, I take my cue from scripture. Matthew 19:4–12 reads,

Have you not read that he who made them from the beginning made them male and female, and said, "For this reason a man shall leave his father and mother and be joined to his wife, and the two shall become one flesh"? So they are no longer two

*but one flesh. What therefore God has joined together, let not man put asunder. They said to him, "Why then did Moses command one to give a certificate of divorce, and to put her away?" He said to them, "For your hardness of heart Moses allowed you to divorce your wives, but from the beginning it was not so. And I say to you: whoever divorces his wife, except for unchastity, and marries another, commits adultery." The disciples said to him, "If such is the case of a man with his wife, it is not expedient to marry." But he said to them, **"Not all men can receive this saying, but only those to whom it is given. For there are eunuchs who have been so from birth, and there are eunuchs who have been made eunuchs by men, and there are eunuchs who have made themselves eunuchs for the sake of the kingdom of heaven. He who is able to receive this, let him receive it."** *(The emphasis is mine.)

This passage doesn't get much press from the pulpit (especially in Republican circles where such political purveyors of "family values" as Bob Dole, Phil Gramm, Pete Wilson, and Newt Gingrich could be convicted of adultery, as specified in the above scripture). However, it is noteworthy because although it acknowledges the sanctity of Heterosexual unions, it is not an injunction to marry. Jesus first explains that God did indeed create two kinds of human beings, female and male (and I would add that we are all a blend of those two elements), and that their union is sacred. He then goes on to explain that not everyone is called to this kind of marriage. He tells us that some people are born "eunuchs," a term from antiquity encompassing a variety of individuals, including those we might today call *Lesbian* or *Gay*.[9]

I interpret this to mean that God makes more kinds of people than just Heterosexuals (*quelle surprise*) and that obviously non-Heterosexuals are not called into a union designed for non-Lavender people. Editors have left us with no further comment, and Jesus seems to offer no specific guidance about how those of us not born Straight might honor our committed relationships. However, the teaching and example of his life clearly indicate that any relationship we enter into with another human being must be just, loving, and honest, and those are actually some pretty good directions right there.

Even though we may not be designed to embrace an institution made for opposite-sex couples, we Lesbians, Gays, and Bisexuals do, however, have the prerogative of taking the only matrimonial blueprint currently available to us and *transforming* it to meet the unique nature of our love relationships by making justice and honesty our priorities.

Now Queer critics of Lesbian and Gay marriage note that we should run faster than Jerry Falwell being chased by RuPaul to escape the trappings of Heterosexual matrimony because of its oppressive history. To most cultures in most times, marriage has been a socially mandated method of controlling women, mainly by confiscating their property, limiting their earning power, and confining them to the parameters of their reproductive functions.

Victoria Brownworth once remarked in a column for *Advocate* magazine that weddings herald misogynist acts worldwide. The brutalities incited by matrimony include battery, rape, and bride-burning. She admonishes same-sex couples not to rush to embrace "this most repressive and repugnant of heterosexual rituals." Although I deem this estimation a bit harsh, though not unfounded, I agree that an institution that has the subjugation of women by men as its original intent ought to have no place in Lavender lives. And although I argue that the Heterosexual marital model is indeed functional in some respects for Homosexuals, I would concede that the metamorphosing of Straight marriage for Lavender folk is additionally dubious because currently it seems to be losing popularity even among Straight people. Heterosexual marriages are dissolving faster than an Alka-Seltzer in water.

In the other critics' corner, Straight scoffers of same-sex unions argue that marriage was designed by God for the purpose of procreation and that, since Lesbians and Gays cannot reproduce, they should not marry. I soundly reject the bogus assumption that Lesbian and Gay pairings cannot foster children. We produce and rear children all the time through artificial insemination and adoption, as well as by coparenting the children a spouse has had by a previous opposite-sex relationship. I further denounce the notion that the right to marry should be contingent upon the willingness or ability of a couple to reproduce. It is a punitive rationale, not to mention inconsistent. I know of no state in the union that denies marriage licenses to infertile opposite-sex couples.

So the only framework for unions presently accessible in American society has some distressing flaws and an abundance of naysayers, but even so, I remain unwilling to chuck the whole concept down the hopper. The joyous public celebration of a sacred obligation and the process of honoring that commitment is vital to a strong society and may be even more important for same-sex couples than for opposite-sex ones because Lesbians and Gays have been told by religion, government, and business that our relationships don't count. But they do. Same-sex unions, like opposite-sex unions, create vital bastions of nurturing and sustenance, which are the firm foundation of any solid social structure. If called, then, Lavender folk must not be dissuaded from marrying.

Of course there are as many ways to create a covenant of love, and the ceremony honoring it, as there are couples to create them.[10] There are also many traditions from which to draw. As Alexah and I learned in designing our own service, even among traditionally andro/anglo/heterocentric rituals there can be found that which is useful. We need not fear brushing too close to the Heterosexual model. We do have plenty of options.

As a recovering alcoholic trying to maintain my sobriety, I have acquired the indispensable art of taking what I like and leaving the rest. It simplifies life and keeps me from getting hung up on trivialities that might impel me to run for the nearest tavern. So, I encourage my Lavender sisters and brothers who are of a mind to marry, not to shun those faith and spiritual traditions with which they are familiar. The chances are that they offer much that is meaningful. What is not readily suitable can be altered, and what is irrelevant can be discarded.

For instance, Alexah and I began crafting our ceremony with "The Celebration and Blessing of a Marriage" found in the Episcopal *Book of Common Prayer.* This particular rite is clearly written for opposite-sex couples, with its numerous references to "this man and this woman," "the union of husband and wife," "united in marriage lawfully," and so on. We decided to deviate substantially from the text, using it only as a guide for the general order of the service, augmenting it with rites from "Covenant Celebration for a Lesbian Couple" in *Women-Church* by Rosemary Radford Ruether.

Rendering the traditionally androcentric, gender-specific language of the liturgy inclusive or gender neutral was a frustrating, but not impossible, process, as was revising the familiar but annoying masculine images of violence and domination so prevalent in scripture.

As another example of turning the Heterosexual caterpillar into a Lavender butterfly, it is customary for the father of the bride to waltz his daughter down the aisle and deposit her safely in the arms of her eagerly awaiting groom. This in effect signifies the transfer of power of one ruling male to another. Clearly such a ritual has no significance for two women. (Besides, as my own father could have attested, he never had any power, real or imagined, over me anyway; so there would have been nothing to transfer.) So we altered this part of the service by inviting my parents and Alexah's chosen parents[11] to share something they had written themselves, thus acknowledging that our union would be bringing two families together as one.

My own mother, drawing up every bit of her feisty 5'2" frame, peered through her Liz Claiborne glasses (with rose-colored frames to match her dress) and pronounced proudly,

> *On this blessed day, we thank God for the gift of Amy in our lives. With her we have laughed and wept. She has brought us growth and joy. Because of her we have learned to see the world and ourselves with new eyes. We loved and nurtured her to the best of our ability, and we taught her to live her own life. As parents, we know we have met our responsibilities well and faithfully because she is able to fly on her own. As Amy moves to a new phase of her life, we send her off with our blessing, knowing that we are not losing a daughter, but instead are gaining one. In the same way that God has shared Amy with us, we now share her with Alexah, and we joyously welcome Alexah into our family of love.*

In addition to overcoming any reticence about drawing from what is familiar, I also encourage Lavender folk to explore lost and suppressed knowledge, traditions, and rituals. Much of the wisdom of our Lesbian, Gay, Bisexual, and Transgendered ancestors has been buried or subverted by centuries of heteropatriarchy. We need to resurrect and reclaim it if we are to exercise our power to name ourselves. Some of the repressed or coopted[12] traditions that we can uncover include Wicca; Sapphic spirit; tribal and indigenous cultures, including the Native-American "two-spirited"[13] and *hwame*[14]; New Age; and dreams, angels, or spirit guides.

As I opined before, marriage, regardless of the tradition on which it is based, must be about love. For me, a foundation of love is not only necessary to my marriage but also to my life as a Christian. That is the reason Alexah and I chose John 13:34 for our service Gospel reading: "*A new commandment I give to you, that you love one another; even as I have loved you, that you also love one another. By this everyone will know that you are my disciples, if you have love for one another.*" I envision that love as warm, affirming, inclusive, and expansive.

The Lavender liberation movement is one of the best things to happen to American society. Lavender lives have helped expand social notions of both marriage and family from rigid, biological definitions that include only a limited number of individuals to ones that make larger connections, helping us see that we are all part of the same human family and that we are accountable to one another. If our world is to learn to open its heart wider in the next millennium, it is essential that Lavender people continue to lead the way by forging marital partnerships and families that allow us all to be loved and cared for. Lesbians, Gays, Bisexuals, and Transgendered people are already constructing matrimonial paradigms that encourage unconditional love, ensure equity, promote integrity, and foster compassion—models in which both partners are accepted as individuals first and are not just defined in terms of each other.

The vows Alexah and I used in our ceremony exemplified these principles well and suited our rather diametric personalities splendidly. Additionally, they confirm my definition of marriage as a bond of love to which both parties must be committed and which must be reaffirmed daily. These poetic vows were written by Kinheart (Wheaton, Illinois), and we adapted them with permission.

Priest: *Do you believe that God has called you both to be witnesses of Christ's love and peace in the world?*

Amy and Alexah: *We do.*

Amy: *Out of all the people and places of my life, it is you with whom I choose to be in special covenant. It is you whom I have chosen to build my life around and with.*[15] *With you I can let my spirit soar. I celebrate the gift of this relationship and the work of giving that gift.*

Alexah: *Of all the people I have known on my journey, it is you with whom I choose to journey on in covenant. With you and your life I choose to weave the strands of my life. I celebrate the gift of this relationship and the work of receiving that gift.*

Amy: *I love you, Alexah, and I want to give you the best of who I am and who I am becoming.*

Alexah: *I choose to live in union with you. I know that the journey may not be easy, but I live better when I live with you.*

Amy: *I promise to work, to play, to dream with you, and to do my best to make those dreams come true.*

Alexah: *I promise to respect you and to celebrate the ways in which you are different from me.*

Amy: *I promise to seek your forgiveness, and forgive you, as we have been forgiven, and I will try with you to better understand ourselves, the world, and God.*

Priest: *You have come here today, in the presence of God, family, and friends, and you have committed your lives to each other. Gracious God, by your holy and life-giving Spirit, pour down upon Alexah and Amy the riches of your grace.*

May the love of Christ draw you into a deep and lasting love for each other, and may your lives together be a continued witness of Christ's love in the world.

By the power of the Holy Spirit, pour out the abundance of your blessings upon Amy and Alexah. Lead them into all peace. Let their love for each other be a seal upon their hearts.

> *Bless them in their work and companionship; in their sleeping and in their waking; in their joys and in their sorrows; in their life and in their death.*
>
> *Finally, in your mercy bring them to that table where your saints feast forever in your heavenly home, through Jesus Christ our Lord, who with you and the Holy Spirit lives and reigns, one God forever.*

Daily, Lavender people enter into similar loving covenants, despite the lack of social or legal affirmation. The status quo as regards societal attitudes and force of law is about to change, however. In which direction, though, remains to be seen.

In May of 1993, the Supreme Court of the State of Hawaii startled the country by ruling that the ban on same-sex marriage violates that state's constitution. In *Baehr v. Lewin* (now *Baehr v. Miike*) the Justices ruled that the state must prove a "compelling state interest" to keep the ban in place. The ruling on a sex discrimination suit brought by three same-sex couples in 1990 set in motion an appeals process that could possibly end with a court decision legalizing same-sex marriage in Hawaii.[16] That decision is expected about the time this anthology is due to publish. No matter what the ruling or its impact on the states, it is still imperative that Lesbians, Gays, Bisexuals, and our Straight allies continue to capitalize on every opportunity to support legally recognized and socially sanctioned marriage between persons of the same sex.

If we learned anything at all from the Gays-in-the-military gaff, we learned from the polls that even among those Americans (including Gay Americans) who normally support Gay rights, those who support Gay marriage are few and far between. No state or federal congressional representative has supported it. Even William Jefferson Clinton, the first president to publicly reserve a place for Lavender people in the White House administration, signed the Defense of Marriage Act dishonoring Gay marriage.

Writing in *Created Equal: Why Gay Rights Matter to America*, Michael Nava and Robert Dawidoff articulate why support for legal same-sex marriage runs so low: "If any one relationship is considered peculiarly heterosexual, it is the marital relationship" (p. 144). No doubt about it, marriage is one of the dominant culture's sacred cows. I think it's a challenge worth taking on, though. Even if we are personally disinclined to marry, it seems in our best interest to support any national campaign to secure the right for same-sex couples to marry. The quality and security of our lives depends on it. Governmental institutions and private industry provide the following perks for legally recognized spouses: the ability to file joint tax returns (which is not always a bonus); joint insurance policies for home, auto, and health benefits; automatic inheritance in the absence of a will; annuities, pension plans, and Social Security and Medicare benefits; veterans' discounts on medical care, education, and home loans; joint custody, adoption, and foster care; wrongful death benefits for a surviving partner and children; bereavement leave when a partner or child dies; and the ability to obtain domestic violence protection orders or divorce protections, such as community property and child support.[17]

Personally, I think that the government has no business approving or disapproving of any love relationship between consenting adults. Like Pat Buchanan, who once said, "We stand with George Bush against the amoral idea that Gay and Lesbian couples should have the same standing in law as [heterosexual] married men and women," the government seems to think that its job is to pass judgment on marital relationships. I don't think the government should grant any couple, same-sex or opposite-sex, entitlements for marrying, but once people are addicted to special favors, it's very hard to withdraw them. I don't see the government butting out. So in the interest of equality, we owe it to ourselves *and to the generations of Lavender youth who will follow us* to secure what Straight people now take for granted.

The fact that Lesbian, Gay, and Bisexual love relationships are not legally sanctioned is an affront to our individual liberty and an insult to our humanity. I remember how disheartened I felt when, a month or two before my own marriage, Alexah and I went to the county courthouse to file for a marriage license. We were curtly told that unless one of us could produce a groom, we would be denied permission to even apply. When we asked why we couldn't fill out the paperwork, we were quoted some inanities from an obscure 20-year-old memo written by the then Recorder of Deeds, who cited precedents from three states other than our own (Missouri) as a legitimate reason why same-sex couples couldn't request a marriage license—unadulterated bullshit. I felt so insignificant. At the same time, though, I was proud that we had the intestinal fortitude to look the heterosexist bureaucrats in the eye and let them know that we're here, we're Queer, and we want to be hitched.

Western culture's heterocentric parameters for couples have inadvertently left us with the notion that any combination of persons besides one woman and one man are somehow suspect, dysfunctional, and inferior. We're uncomfortable, even hostile, to the concept and reality of same-sex couples. It's disconcerting to contemplate same-sex marriages because we get a migraine trying to figure out who's the "wife" and who's the "husband."[18]

This naturally brings me to the final but extremely important matter of language, a powerful means of communication that springs directly from our belief systems and shapes our everyday reality. No discussion of Lavender identity, relationships, or equality would be complete without it.

You'll notice that many terms associated with traditional opposite-sex lifestyles are encumbered by gender associations. These words are products of a culture that defines women and men only in terms of each other and reflects the cultural obsession with sex. As Alexah and I learned from trying to write a wedding ceremony, such a lopsided focus has left our vocabulary sadly bereft of images, concepts, and definitions for same-sex couples and their families. As Victoria Brownworth once put it, "We have gone from 'the love that dare not speak its name'[19] to the love that doesn't know its name."

The following Lavender lingo constitutes just a few of the many possibilities for naming the families we have created by *choice* and not by *chance*.

Opposite-sex term: *Wife, husband*

Same-sex counterpart: *Life-partner, lover, spouse, mate, soul-mate, life-mate, significant other, partner, domestic partner*

Comment: Alexah and I do not recommend the term *lover*. Even though the root is *love*, it conjures up images of a purely sexual relationship or else a sexual relationship that involves affection but no commitment of the soul. Although some opposite-sex marriages may be purely physical in that they are for reproductive purposes only, same-sex relationships can be deeper than that. All this, of course, is not to say that sex is a bad thing.

We also do not favor the term *partner* because it is somewhat ambiguous, suggesting a purely business-type arrangement. *Significant other* doesn't really fill the bill either because it sounds like some sort of statistical average.

We're not terribly fond of *domestic partner,* at least in the familial sense, because it makes us sound like house pets. However, in the corporate and legal sense, it is a functional phrase and a crucial concept. It is important to note that the term *domestic partner* applies to same-sex couples as well as to unmarried opposite-sex couples not yet considered married by common law. Actually, an even newer designation is coming into vogue—*spousal equivalent.* Sounds like the generic form of the brand name, doesn't it?

Our personal favorite is *life-partner.* The major drawback to this term is that it has too many syllables. Life-mate might actually be a better choice, since it has one less syllable for the tongue to get around.

Opposite-sex term: *Wedding*
Same-sex counterpart: *Holy union, joining, covenant, marriage, wedding*
Comment: Although many groups and individuals, religious and nonreligious, quibble over whether "wedding" can properly be used to describe the union of a same-sex couple, Alexah and I say, "Of course it can, silly, if you want it to."

Opposite-sex term: *Mother, father*
Same-sex counterpart: *Parent, coparent, mother, father*
Comment: *Coparent,* though somewhat foreign to the ear, is my personal favorite because it implies an equity and cooperation in childrearing, which is sadly missing from heterocentric definitions.

Opposite-sex term: *Mother-in-law, father-in-law, daughter-in-law, son-in-law*
Same-sex counterpart: *Mother-in-love, father-in-love, daughter-in-love, son-in-love*
Comment: You astute readers have already figured out that the operative principle here is to substitute "love" for "law." Although I favor the legalization of same-sex marriage, I still prefer this

substitution, since it suggests that our families are authorized by love rather than by some bureaucratic governmental seal of approval.

Opposite-sex term: *Family*
Same-sex counterpart: *Chosen family*
Comment: *Family* in the heteropatriarchal context really means "family of origin," or the group of individuals with whom you share your DNA. Alexah and I are very committed to the concept of *chosen family.* This term suggests a conscious choice in creating those vital bastions of love and nurturing, rather than some haphazard biological accident.

We are, without a doubt, the product of our experiences, and as an adopted child, I have lived for nearly 40 years with the knowledge that I was undoubtedly the inconvenient result of a few moments of hormonal hoopla on someone's couch one night. In addition to my sexual orientation, my status as an adoptee makes me that much more zealous in my assertion that we must be responsible, thoughtful, and prayerful in our creation of families.

Although standardizing our nomenclature might help us be more articulate and cohesive (and as my mother once suggested, it would help give Straight people a clue), we probably ought not to box ourselves in too tightly, thereby leaving our options open. That is, after all, what the Lesbian, Gay, Bisexual, and Transgendered liberation movement is all about—broadening our horizons, expanding our notions and options, including more people, and encouraging people not to limit themselves or marginalize others. There is perhaps no greater power in the world than the power to choose, welcome, love, and affirm.

NOTES

1. Contrary to the immutable rules of English grammar, I choose to capitalize most adjectives and nouns identifying sexual orientation, especially variant orientations. It is my way of acknowledging their importance without overemphasizing it.

2. A term of endearment for fundamentalist Christians, who account for the largest faction of the theocratic juggernaut, which is attempting to dismantle the constitutional separation between Church and State and impose one narrowly prescribed set of "Christian" values on America, a multicultural democracy.

3. I often use the term *Lavender* rather than *Queer* to encompass the spectrum of sexual minority lives, e.g., Lesbian, Gay, Bisexual, Transgendered, Transsexual, Transvestite, Butch, Femme, and Gender-Variant. The quest to find suitable terminology to define ourselves is part of the liberation process. Although I sometimes use the word *Queer* as shorthand, I prefer Lavender because it is more beautiful and has a less contentious linguistic history. The word Lavender as a description for sexual minorities is not an original creation. Occasionally, I use the word *Homosexual* to describe persons with a same-sex orientation, but I only use it for the sake of variety. I find it far too clinical for common usage.

4. A pathological fear of same-sex intimacy and eroticism, homophobia is rooted in sexism, or the fear and negation of the feminine. It should not be confused with the related but different term *heterosexism*, which is the assumption or presumption that everyone is or should be Heterosexual. Heterosexism is implicit in all American institutions, including marriage.

5. The texts of terror include a mere half dozen or so passages lifted from both the Hebrew and Christian scriptures. It is notable that none of them are taken from the Gospels. These scriptures are used to justify denying sexual minorities the same civil rights (e.g., equal access to housing, employment, public accommodations, privacy, and health care coverage) that are accorded the sexual majority. They are also used to justify the outright execution of Lavender people. These intentionally misconstrued texts usually include Genesis 19; Leviticus 18:22 and 20:13; Deuteronomy 23:17, 18; Romans 1:18–32; I Corinthians 6:9; and I Timothy 1:10.

6. John 8:15.

7. Two consenting adults, that is, who are not related by blood. Even though incest is modeled nicely for us in Genesis, I do not consider it a component for a healthy marriage.

8. Alexah and I used to joke with each other that the vows were valid only until the good times were over or the money ran out—whichever came first.

9. I refer readers to a fine discourse on Lavender people in antiquity written by Rev. Nancy Wilson in *Our Tribe: Queer Folks, God, Jesus, and the Bible.* HarperSanFrancisco, 1995.

10. I refer readers to the following excellent resources: *Equal Rites: Lesbian and Gay Worship, Ceremonies, and Celebrations,* edited by Kittredge Cherry and Zalmon Sherwood (Westminster John Knox Press, 1995); *Ceremonies of the Heart: Celebrating Lesbian Unions,* edited by Becky Butler (Seal Press, 1990); and *The Essential Guide to Lesbian and Gay Weddings,* by Tess Ayers and Paul Brown (HarperSanFrancisco, 1994).

11. Alexah's biological parents were present at our wedding but chose not to participate in the service because they do not approve of our relationship. In their absence, not only from the service but also from their daughter's life, Alexah asked Ann and Charlie Watts, a wonderful Heterosexual couple from our parish, to stand in as her parents. See also the discussion of "Lavender lingo" on pp. 92-94.

12. Remember that the seasons of the Christian calendar, such as Lent and Advent, as well as many of its holy days, such as Easter and Christmas, have been coopted from the worship of the Goddess at the spring and winter solstice.

13. "Two-spirited" refers to morphological male who has a nontraditional social role and may have a special ceremonial role. He performs some women's work and blends much of the behavior and dress of women and men.

14. Hwame are Lesbian cross-dressers, considered among the Mojave to be shamans.

15. Recalling these words in jest, I once told Alexah, "Out of all the people and places in my life, you are the least dysfunctional. Therefore, I choose you!"

16. In anticipation of a favorable ruling for same-sex couples from the Hawaii Supreme Court, several states introduced legislation defining marriage as something that may only take place between a man and woman. Such legislation is revoltingly reminiscent of miscegenation laws, which, until as recently as the 1960s, forbade marriage between blacks and whites.

17. This list was taken from *Freedom to Marry: Key Questions and Answers*, a pamphlet produced by The Gay and Lesbian Alliance Against Defamation, (212) 807–1700.

18. This points to one of the obvious conveniences of opposite-sex marriages, which is the already specified gender-based division of labor. She does the laundry, and he takes out the garbage. Of course, my own marriage has been a breeze because I do the laundry and put out the trash.

19. Said by Oscar Wilde, referring to Homosexuality.

Chapter 7

Variety Is the Spice of Life
Doing It Our Ways

Mary E. Hunt

Although some may wish to live coupled, what about those who, regardless of sexual identity, are single by choice or chance, those who find three or four a more congenial pattern, those who prefer community? Perpetuating the marriage model for yet more people seems to be perpetuating a double standard in favor of those who partner at the expense of those who do not.

Women in general have fared poorly in marriage, even worse in divorce, hence my feminist urge for a little relational creativity. After all, the trend toward individualism is only detoured by coupledom, not rerouted toward community as I think it should be. A married person is still only one person away from being single, just as so many women are one man away from welfare.

Normative sexuality for my Roman Catholic parents was heterosexual sex open to as many children as the Lord would send. Family was Mom, Dad, and the three children, duly sent. Normative sex for me is lesbian love expressed safely and with the hope that my partner and I both enjoy it. Family is myself, my lover, and our "significant multitude"—friends and blood relatives with whom we share life. How times change.

Times have changed because of birth control, the AIDS pandemic, and population concerns. So my parents' norm seems almost medieval to my generation. Likewise, lots of different relational constellations compose families now, especially in urban areas where large numbers of lesbian, gay, bisexual, and transgendered people live. Yet times have not really changed much since there seems to be a tendency toward maintaining a normative position, "the way it is done," a monolithic approach, even though it differs from that of a previous generation. *The result is that seemingly progressive efforts like same-sex marriages can be coopted into forming* the *new norm, effectively preventing relational variety, and implicitly dividing the "good gays" from the "bad gays."* I submit that we are better off, though not much, for having the newly emerging norm, but that we will be much better off only when we can make the world safe for variety.

In this essay I explore the theme of same-sex marriages as an example of something new quickly becoming normative. I will focus on the right of queer folk to celebrate our love, friendship, and commitment as we see fit, as well as the need to foster variety for *all* of our survival at a time of right-wing backlash.

I write as a theologian interested in questions of meaning and value. I live in a long-term relationship, but have not celebrated it publicly in either the religious or the legal realm.

The nicest wedding I ever attended was in a Quaker meeting house, followed by a swish reception with two lavender brides on the top of a double chocolate wedding cake. The service was taste-ful—Quaker silence and well-chosen words. One participant remarked during the time for congregational comments that Annie, one of the brides, was "the reason for a smile of uncommon radiance on the face of Lynnae (the other bride)." I quite agreed. They have lived happily ever after, amen.

Many of us could tell lovely tales by now of same-sex weddings we have attended. In the face of breast cancer and AIDS epidemics in our communities, public commitments are a good way to express our care before it is all over. This is a human right that needs to be recognized as such.

The economic and social ramifications, the changes that will have to be made as such ceremonies take on legal significance, are important. Fair is fair; married is married. But in candor and justice, there is another side to all of this, which deserves exploration, lest we romanticize ourselves into a corner.

Some celebrations have been videotaped, with the tape lasting longer than the relationship. Others have been painful affairs with hurt over parental rejection exacerbated by family members unwill-ing to attend the ceremony. Still others have never gone beyond the discussion stage, with intimacy issues surfacing and old tapes rolling about what marriage means, to the extent that folks have bailed out of the whole relationship. Love is like that sometimes. In all, I suspect that the ups and downs of wedded bliss accrue to lesbian, gay, bisexual, and transgendered people in roughly equal measure to our heterosexual counterparts, albeit with that extra hassle deriving from the fact that we are not "supposed" to marry.

The extra measure is not incidental, nor trivial, but neither should overcoming it be the sole goal as we reshape the world to make space for ourselves. My goal is to make love abound in a world where there is precious little of it and to make love fair. Insofar as same-sex marriages do that, I applaud them. But if they simply make the world a little more convenient for some people while still leaving others aside, I am less than enthusiastic.

Recently, my partner and I bought a new car. My partner's name and not mine had been on the title for our previous car, since I had been too lazy to brave the Department of Motor Vehicles' lines. When it came time to transfer the license plates, the salesperson just wrote it up with both of our names. But when the man who collected our savings account in exchange for the car noted the discrepancy, he announced that we had to pay another fee. If we had been married, the transfer would have been free. Even the car salesman understood and sympathized when we argued that if we had been married for a week instead of partnered for 15 years we could have gone out for dinner instead of writing another check. In short, it is not such a stretch for most people to see the injustice perpetrated by the marriage norm.

The question is how best to get beyond it. Issues like inheritance, visiting rights, powers of attorney, immigration, and the like are very real and very expensive compared with the streamlined way in which marriage conveys certain rights. The debate over whether or not to wed is a sign of how far we have come as lesbian, gay, bisexual, and transgendered people. That some of the same churches that have rejected us are entertaining the notion seriously makes me alternately delighted and skeptical. In a nutshell, as long as certain rights and responsibilities accrue to those heterosexuals who marry, I believe that these same things should accrue to lesbian and gay people as well. *But as long as lesbian and gay people have a choice,*

I urge us to take leadership in breaking the two-by-two pattern that is alleged to have begun with Noah and his nameless wife.

Although some may wish to live coupled, what about those who, regardless of sexual identity, are single by choice or chance, those who find three or four a more congenial pattern, those who prefer community? Perpetuating the marriage model for yet more people seems to be perpetuating a double standard in favor of those who partner at the expense of those who do not.

Women in general have fared poorly in marriage, even worse in divorce, hence my feminist urge for a little relational creativity. After all, the trend toward individualism is only detoured by coupledom, not rerouted toward community as I think it should be. A married person is still only one person away from being single, just as so many women are one man away from welfare.

My own view is that friendship and not coupledness ought to be the relational norm, if there must be one. I have argued that the heterosexual marriage norm is inadequate for the needs of most people and that it should be replaced by friendship.[1] At least friendships are always plural, and one can choose to befriend oneself or one's cat and still be considered within the realm. This Jesuit approach to getting away from a normative approach is really a call to variety. I issue it to keep the discussion going, lest we bypass an opportunity to make substantive structural changes and not just the, comparatively speaking, cosmetic changes that same-sex marriages will be.

It is hard to argue against what seems to be a step forward for lesbian and gay people. In fact, I believe that the *right* to marry is essential to our full inclusion in society. After all, if social legitimacy is conferred this way and stability enhanced, who am I to nix it? Further, if children are to be brought into our homes with some semblance of security, perhaps marriage is a good start. Even more convincing to some religious people is the sacramental grace of marriage. In its best guise, it is the prayerful support of a loving community that is brought to bear on a given twosome. If weddings are really excuses to celebrate and share the wealth, who would look the collective gift horse in the mouth? Although I am not unalterably opposed to such practices, I do find that they reinscribe patriarchal norms with ever more virulence against those who choose not to conform.

I have seen real good come out of such ceremonies, like the healing of family bonds or the mixing of various communities. Still, I have strong reservations and suggest that we ponder the ins and outs before the wedding industry closes in around us. Capitalism and the nuclear family will be happily bolstered by more adherents of which I am loath to become one.

For all of their benefits, lesbian and gay marriage ceremonies do three things that give me pause. First, they focus on couples at a time when I think community needs emphasis. Two people need support to maintain and deepen a relationship. But especially for lesbian women, though I think also for gay men, the need to build strong networks of friends, an extensive and intensive support system within which to live, a safety net within which to fall, seems equally important. Why not celebrate that instead of or in addition to a coupled relationship?

For example, a friend who was moving invited all of her women friends to send her forth. It was a time to say what she meant to us, to wish her well, and to promise a permanent presence in her life even though she would be far away. Nothing about a commitment service precludes our doing this; but if the norm is a wedding, it will take great imagination to see this kind of option and to take it seriously as an important expression of commitment.

Coupled relationships are as much an economic covenant as an emotional one. Whether joint checking accounts, life insurance beneficiaries, or other niceties of advanced capitalism, coupled relationships reinforce the notion of "just the two of us against the world," which helps to keep the wheels of the system running. I suspect that advanced patriarchal capitalism can stand a few same-sex couples here and there, especially in the top economic brackets. But most of us would be better off if we socialized our resources. Why reinforce the economic and social mode that has kept so many people down if we have a choice? Our whole way of thinking in twos and/or nuclear families mitigates against such social creativity just when those on the bottom of the economic heap need it most.

I was struck by the reaction among a group of lesbian professionals, many of whom enthusiastically raised their hands in response to the question of whether they were or wanted to be married. Of course, at the upper income levels much more is permitted, but the question is what its implications are for those at the bottom. Likewise, the lesbian/gay wedding discussion seems to be a predominantly white phenomenon. What are the class and race assumptions that make it such? And what is there to learn from people for whom it is not an economic or social option?

Second, same-sex coupling services reinforce the notion that relationships are forever and ever, amen. Heterosexual marriages were styled this way, and as politically correct as the wording may be, the same-sex covenants I have witnessed have had that "forever" quality of which I am increasingly suspicious. It is not that I encourage promiscuity or reject stability. It is simply that I wonder if quantity (i.e., forever) and not quality (i.e., while it is healthy, life-giving, and community-enhancing for both persons) is really the issue when it comes to love. Heterosexual people with their 50 percent divorce rate have discovered that longer life spans have made "forever" a relative term.

Will commitment services encourage people (women especially, who sometimes stay together long after it would have been healthy to split) to persevere in a rocky relationship because it has been celebrated publicly? Will the partners feel constrained by their commitment to share their struggles with people who could help because the wedding created an illusion about the perfect couple? Perhaps it will work the other way, and another married couple will be able to help precisely because they do understand. But where does this leave folks who live together without the benefit of a ceremony?

The larger point is that many problems that couples have stem from placing too much emotional freight on one relationship, missing the fact that we need many people with whom to interact, indeed to love, in order to meet our myriad relational needs.

Third, if covenants were to become the norm within our communities, what does this mean about those of us who live, albeit some of us in monogamous, committed relationships, without benefit of such celebrations? Will we become the new "unwed mothers" and couples "living in sin"? Far-fetched as this may sound, I reject any move toward neopuritanism that will gain lesbian, gay, bisexual, and transgendered love respectability by mimicking the heterosexual model. I take every opportunity to cheer for variety in our relational lives.

Likewise, I wonder whether some of the urge toward same-sex commitment services isn't part of an unconscious move to make us OK; to sanitize our love, which needs no such soap and water; to mainstream us when in fact the mainstream needs a good push in the direction of honesty. After all, heterosexual variety is the legacy of the 1960s, and from all accounts it is a lasting legacy. Indeed, some elderly people now opt for living together rather than losing Social Security and other retirement benefits from their deceased spouses when they repartner. Granted, the system "works" for them, but it strikes me that the goal is to make it work for everyone, not just for a few more who conform to the prevailing model.

The heterosexual community has much to learn from us. We have much to teach: our strong reliance on one another for survival, not simply on our partner, if we have one, but on our community; life with dignity and fun even if we are not partnered; endless variety in how we make our lives work in the face of oppression. These are valuable contributions that, when taken seriously, will reshape the ethical norms of our society.

Same-sex commitment ceremonies are increasingly common. They are a regular part of some churches, such as the Metropolitan Community Church and other reasonable religious groups that take love seriously. Far from wanting to put an end to them, I urge that we expand their scope, widen their parameters, and begin to see how communal and personal lives can be enhanced when such supportive ceremonies are made available to everyone whether coupled or not. Croning ceremonies, or rites of passage, for older women are a good example of the variety of rituals that mark more than one-to-one relationships.

My beginning exploration of options is meant to complement that movement so that we can turn the oppression of heterosexist patriarchy into the liberation of friends. John Boswell's book, *Same-Sex Unions in Premodern Europe,* has brought this question to public attention through Doonesbury cartoons and the most erudite scholarly debates.[2] Boswell established the basis for, if not the definitive proof of, the existence of some ceremonies in premodern Europe, which lifted same-sex love to public expression. Whether these were marriages as such and whether or not they were precursors of the present-day same-sex commitment ceremonies is the question.

Think of your dearest friends, the ones whom you call "family of choice," the ones without whom life would be meaningless. Think of far-flung friends, old friends, and work and work-out colleagues with whom you have become closer over the years, a neighbor who has become a real mainstay, or your sister or brother who has surprised you over the years by her or his love. The list is endless and so are the celebrations—parties, liturgies, an annual picnic, Thanksgiving at home, your birthday. The form is not as important as the content, and the content is honest love, not just for one other but for several, many, perhaps in the next life for all.

Unfortunately in our communities we have become all too accustomed to going to funerals. AIDS and breast cancer have taken so many of our peers, so many premature deaths. Why not move from the reflexive same-sex unions to the community-enhancing and structure-changing celebrations that will include more than simply couples, and more than people who are dead? I encourage variety without in any way stopping the wedding music.

The main reason I encourage this is that the powerful influence of right-wing backlash ensures that things will not change much for any of us if it does not change some for all of us. The misnamed religious right leads the way with out-and-out homo-hatred, which translates into making us (along with other unpopular groups, such as welfare moms) the enemy that takes the place of Communists after the end of the Cold War. A few of us may be able to get by, but most of us, especially poor people and people of color, already on the social periphery, are in real danger.

The twistings of the religious right are so profound as to have us biologically identified women and men divided from one another. Lesbian women, in their imaginations, are consigned to a literal no-man's-land where the right imagines we ride our motorcycles and seduce their children. Gay men are forever fornicating, in their dreams of course. But with the media money of the so-called right, such images are implanted in the public psyche with little resistance. This is not homophobia but hatred and malice toward us; nor is it as religious as it is political, which is why I will not concede the misnomer "religious right." It is into this background that so many well-intentioned among us reason that if we can just be as good, read "monogamous," as they want, all will be well. I doubt it, with ample bashing and job losses in our communities to confirm my intuition.

Even if it were true that some couples were socially, that is economically and politically, "acceptable," what does it mean for the rest of us? I suggest that contrary to our hopes, it will mean that the same charges of promiscuity, perversion, and worse will accrue to those who do not measure up, with our new norms contributing to our oppression. Never mind that our dating and divorce patterns will mirror heterosexuals. *It will always be our sexual identity and not our relational fortunes that matter until and unless we break the hegemony of marriage.*

We have learned some lessons from years of right-wing backlash. We have learned to reject categorically their portrayals of us and to stay as close to the texts of our own lives as we can to keep our own equilibrium and prevent others from setting the agenda for us. Those texts are varied and diverse; there is no such thing as "the gay community." There are only many groupings and enclaves, many friends and communities that do their best to survive.

The way it works in our society is that the right-wing is capable of absorbing a few of us who are white enough, wealthy enough, professional enough, monogamous enough to fit into their schema. But they will use some of us as a wedge against the rest of us. Just because my partner and I are beyond our seventeenth anniversary and are white professionals who own a house and can pay the neighbor boy to keep the lawn cut, I do not want to be used, however unwittingly, as a tool to deprive my sister or brother, my gay, queer, bi, and trans friends of their relational freedom. This is what it means to live in solidarity in vicious times.

Variety is practical for its own sake as well. After all, anything can happen in a relationship, and most of us will live long enough to have several relational experiences after leaving the blood or adoptive family of our early years. This is especially the case for the many heterosexually married people who find themselves coming out in marriage. Some choose to maintain their marriage (often for the children's sake just like so many heterosexual people) and to have same-sex relationships at the same time. Others among us choose serial monogamy, or just never find a person with whom partnership is desired. Yet more lesbian, gay, bisexual, and transgendered people lose their partners to death. In short, life is too complicated for easy solutions like same-sex marriage as the new panacea, and we are too varied to make it the new norm. So while there is still time, before the right pushes us into an ill-fitting respectability, I urge that we keep the relational options open and fluid for the foreseeable future.

NOTES

1. Mary E. Hunt. *Fierce Tenderness: A Feminist Theology of Friendship.* New York: Crossroad, 1991.

2. John Boswell. *Same-Sex Love in Premodern Europe.* New York: Vintage Books, 1994.

Chapter 8

The Transforming Power of Queer Love

Brad Wishon

It is the challenge of having to "leave one's father and mother behind" in the choice of a mate that is teaching us to build new "families of choice." This creates a paradigm wherein heterosexuals are learning from queers how to survive in a migratory society. It is the challenge of having to build a life in the face of death and disease that is teaching us to experience life, rather than to just let life happen. This creates a fundamental shift in the way heterosexuals view their partnerships. It is ceasing to be about continuing the tribe and becoming a way of loving and nurturing others to reach their potential. Relationship becomes nurture, not transaction; support, not supply.

═══════════

I believe in the holiness, the sanctity, of love, whatever flavor it might be—gay, lesbian, bisexual, transgendered, heterosexual, or other. Because I believe in love, I want to do all I can to help love flourish. In that process I have been party to everything from proceding down gold mylar "aisles" through fog machines in a candle-lit sanctuary to recessing to Billy Idol's "White Wedding." I have presided over ceremonies in bars, in churches, in the park, in homes, at gardens, and in hotel suites. I have celebrated weddings where the attire of the day was jeans, tuxedos, custom designs, and fringed leather. I have been a party to both elaborate dramas and simple exchanges of the words "I love you," all because I believe in the holiness of love, including queer love.

It is my observation that we are, in fact, changing the face of primary relationships in the United States, and it is reflected in large part by our celebration ceremonies. The celebration of queer love begins in much the same way as heterosexual love. One partner decides to ask the other to make a unique commitment beyond the pledge of "I love you." It is done in informal settings, at romantic dinners, at exotic vacation spots, and in the privacy of the bedroom. But it is a bigger step than the one taken by a heterosexual couple. It is the biggest risk one might ever take in life. The queer ceremony is considered immoral by most of the people the couple encounters in life. To propose such a thing, or agree to it, is to invite the scorn of those who hate queers.

Such a process could be compared with "coming out" for gay, lesbian, bisexual, and transgendered folk. Just as a person who is queer eventually begins to reveal that truth to others, sometimes in small ways, sometimes in a **big** way, so do queer couples go through a process of "coming out." That process can be one of affirmation and growth, but most often it is a process of discovering who will accept you as long as you don't "practice" your love. Much of society believes that queer folk should bury their heads in the "relationship" sands and ignore love. Yet when gay men are found in parks ignoring relational love but fulfilling physical need, they are criticized. *There is no way to appease irrational bias, thus we must work to erode its control on society.*

By its very nature then, the celebration of queer love is a risk we take to do justice. It is to reach out beyond the constraints of society's need to order itself in familiar ways. We go beyond just living together and pretending to be "roommates," and state that two people believe their love is holy. Thus, the celebration takes on a very different quality—so much so that a straight photographer who works with me will decline to shoot a heterosexual wedding to do work for a queer holy union. She does this because there is something about the celebration that goes beyond an "ordinary wedding," and because there is a certain holiness and beauty of the queer ceremony, which resonates within this photographer in ways she often does not find in heterosexual marriages. The holy union is not only an awesome statement of love and respect but also *a demand for justice.*

In the United States today any two people who consider a life together face the challenges of finances, careers, children, family obligations, and future shifts in relational desires. But two queer folk considering life together face all of these and more. There is social stigma to be dealt with. There is the threat of AIDS among gay men and bisexual males and the threat of tripled incidence of breast cancer among lesbians and bisexual women. There is the risk of losing one's career because of one's so-called lifestyle or loss of family for the same reason. However, it is precisely these elements of queer family building and the celebration of queer love that are reshaping society's ways of being in relationship.

It is the challenge of having to "leave one's father and mother behind" in the choice of a mate that is teaching us to build new "families of choice." This creates a paradigm wherein heterosexuals are learning from queers how to survive in a migratory society. It is the challenge of having to build a life in the face of death and disease that is teaching us to experience life, rather than to just let life happen. This creates a fundamental shift in the way heterosexuals view their partnerships. It is ceasing to be about continuing the tribe and becoming a way of loving and nurturing others to reach their potential. Relationship becomes nurture, not transaction; support, not supply.

In this shift, queer folk are leading the way out of the paradigm of transactional relationship, wherein the man gets a cleaning service, a cook, a nanny, and sexual satisfaction, and the woman gets an income, a home, a caregiver, and sexual satisfaction. The shift leads to a paradigm of relationship based on mutuality. In the end, it is mutuality that relationship is about—nurturing and caring to facilitate growth—though this is not to imply that this has not happened in heterosexual relationships before this period in our history. It has, but not as a result of existing paradigms of relationship. Rather, it has happened, often in spite of the form of relationship predominant in society. This is not so in queer relationship. The old structures, by and large, do not work. Therefore a change in the way we create relationship is mandated by the very nature of queer relationship, and it is affecting the world.

We see it in the role women now play in society. A woman is no longer required to surrender her family name upon marrying. She can choose to keep it, combine it with her mate's name, or surrender to the old traditions that tell her she does not have an identity separate from a man. In that old view, she either carries her father's or husband's name; but without connection to a man, she does not exist.

I believe more and more women are choosing to exist apart from men as a result of the shifts being produced by queer love. In its very essence, queer love challenges the old notions of patriarchal domination. Queer love goes beyond the barriers erected by a male-dominated society—for female and male queers alike—because it necessitates a relationship that is not about profit but about nurture.

In queer relationship celebrations you may yet find the old elements of vows, music, rings, candles, all the niceties that say "I love you." What you will not find are the transactional properties of many heterosexual weddings. No one "gives" anyone away. An individual is offering her or his love to another, both with mutual power, dignity, and choice. In queer celebrations, no one agrees to obey anyone, and no one changes status. One person does not surrender prior identity to assume her or his partner's.

The relationship model shifts from property to personhood, and with it, the resultant need to become more open to different ways of being in relationship. *I believe the heterosexual divorce rate in the United States is as high as it is because society is not allowing divergent ways of being in relationship to enter the mainstream.* Thus, the only recourse to changes in a relationship is to end it. Relationship is not static, it is human and therefore fluid. So its institutions and structures must be fluid as well.

Very often we hear of late-term divorces, in which a man and woman have been married for 15 to 20 years, raised children, and then divorced. There are many theories that float around as to what happens; for example, interests change; or life goals are different. There seem to be very few responses, outside of divorce, to the problem, though. Is it possible that the other options available are just too uncomfortable for us to discuss? These might include celibate marriages, open relationships, marriages where the partners live separately during parts of the year. These are happening, but we are not talking about them. Thus, we continue to see the wasteland of lives left behind in the wake of nasty separations and divorces.

In addition to women retaining their birthnames and relationships assuming a less transactional tone, one of the more concrete ways we see the celebration of queer love changing the paradigms of human relationship is in corporate structures. Corporations are a reflection of society. There are now numerous companies, many of them Fortune 500 companies—for example, Lotus, Apple, IBM, and Disney—that extend benefits to employees' chosen, but not legal, spouses and families. I believe one of the key factors in this is the very presence of queer celebrations of love, made prominent through the simplest of ways; for instance, an invitation to the supervisor, a request for time off to prepare for the ceremony or for leisure time following it, a mention of a partner's birthday or some special occasion. All of these give employers clues about their employees lives and how they need to make sure their employees are cared for.

Queer folk are changing the face of relationship in the United States merely by presenting other faces of relationship. We do it most frequently when we celebrate our love. Sometimes the celebration is loud and vibrant, with much fanfare. Other times it is subtle, quiet, and dignified. But always, it is a celebration of love that bit by bit is changing the face of relationship. The impact of it is only now beginning to surface.

The recent resurgence of extremist views opposing the common ground shared by most Americans on abortion, gun control, welfare, and other social issues is in direct opposition to the shifts in relationship happening today. So it is not hard to understand why queer folk have been targeted so vehemently by theocratic smear campaigns. It is queer folk who are at the forefront of these monumental societal shifts. So the very appearance of relationship outside of a transactional concept will bring down swift retribution from the theocratic thought police who seek to eradicate all forms of relationship except their own.

What I find most amazing in this entire spectacle is that even the organizations that biblical literalists have built to defeat the "gay agenda" are being forced to change because society is made up of more people who do not fit their mold than those who do. They are being forced by natural evolution to incorporate people into their organizations who are in family groupings that are not the "perfect family unit," all the while they are seeking to stop those same changes from continuing. Religious and social institutions can no longer bury their heads in the sand and ignore divorce, single-parent families, and extended family arrangements, for these make up the majority of relationships in the United States today. All the while extremist religious groups are denouncing these paradigms, they are slowly evolving within their own organizations to accommodate the differences that are present by the very nature of humanity. Humans will be a part of their society. Within their organizations they are slowly, sometimes microscopically, being compelled to accommodate single parents, working women, and minority cultures and traditions. Queer erosion of the elusive relationship ideal they propose is even affecting the very organizations seeking to eradicate queer love.

In queer love today we find then that we are learning how to "build" families, rather than inherit them. We are discovering ways to give birth to or adopt children. We are making our families visible, obvious, and a part of the fabric of our communities, from New York City to Paducah.

In my own life, I have come to experience this societal shift. Its impact has been of a very personal nature. Two years ago, my life-mate and I celebrated our holy union in a church, with a pastor presiding, people praying, songs being sung, music being played, children laughing, and mothers crying. It sounds so ordinary.

It is, however, anything but ordinary. Our experience with our families was vastly different from our siblings' experiences were with them for their weddings. We were forced to "explain" the ceremony. We were asked repeatedly why it was necessary. We were sent letters telling us that although we were loved, we were sinners that needed forgiveness because we loved each other and sought to celebrate this great gift we have been given in one another. However, because we sent invitations to family members, they now must acknowledge both of us in cards, greetings, and visits. There can be no separation of us in their minds ever again.

Our holy union changed the way we relate not only to relatives, but also to people we work with. It's hard to miss the ring on the "marriage" finger. And we will never lie and disavow our love for each other. People we encounter professionally and socially who are brave enough to ask, hear of the love of two men for each other and how that love called for a sacred and celebratory commitment.

Our union has certainly impacted my ecumenical work. As a pastor, I serve on a variety of ecumenical and interfaith boards. I was already very open about my sexual orientation, but our holy union made that even more prominent. These folks are my colleagues, my co-workers in service. I could not simply avoid inviting them, nor did I wish to. So we invited them to attend our celebration, and many of them came. There were elders, pastors, deacons, rabbis, and priests; some with their wives, husbands, and partners; others alone; and still others with their families in tow. All of them had come to witness the love between two men, celebrated in a holy union. One ceremony has touched hundreds of lives.

Queer celebrations of love are changing the world. Thousands of times each year we are stepping out to declare the holiness of our love, to celebrate the value of our love, and to elevate our bonds and our families. And thousands of times we are creating changes that are shifting all of society's views of relationships. Who knows? In a few short centuries, someone may be trying to uncover the roots of relationship celebrations. They will be amazed to find out that there was a time when only certain forms of love were condoned. Even more amazing will be the revelation that the healthiest views of relationship were born out of celebrations that the society of this day called *immoral*. The sands of relationship are shifting, and the power behind the shift is queer love.

Chapter 9

Together on the Path
Gay Relationships in a Buddhist Context

Michael J. Sweet

Throughout almost all of its history, in the many cultures in which it flourished, Buddhism has profoundly rejected what the benighted American right-wing calls "traditional family values." The basic paradigm is found in the life story of Sākyamuni, the Buddha (Awakened One). He was a very sheltered, upper-class young man, who was already married with a young son, when his first view of sick, aging, and dead people took away his pleasure in family life, and the sight of a homeless mendicant gave him hope of a way out. For Sākyamuni, no less than for the Jesus of the Gospels, the biological family was an impediment to spiritual growth, to be left behind if necessary.

Lenny and I had been together for three years when he went to live in a Buddhist monastery. He didn't promise to return, and I was devastated, feeling I had lost the best thing that had ever happened in my life. We had met at a classic Queer venue of the pre-Stonewall era, the fabled standees' line of the old Metropolitan Opera on Eighth Avenue[1] It didn't happen totally by chance. The go-between was my old high-school friend, Phil, a slightly closeted Irish Catholic who had met this "interesting and acerbic Jew" at Fordham and thought that we must be meant for each other. He was right! The meeting was like a thunderclap of good fortune—an attractive guy my age, who was brainy, witty, and musical. We hit it off immediately, and he invited me to visit him in farthest Rockaway to see his Oscar Wilde collection—this sounded promising. I wasn't sure if he was gay, nor did he know I was, but we immediately formed a very close friendship and spent all the time we could together. We whiled away the hours listening to Bach and Wagner, reciting Baudelaire and Swinburne, walking drunkenly through the city, talking endlessly, and finally one fine spring morning falling into each other's arms with long-suppressed desire. This was in the mid-1960s, in an America still intensely homophobic, with few openly gay couples in evidence to serve as role models. I knew there was a gay subculture in New York, but imagined it in unappealing terms—bitchy, swishy, superficial, and alcoholic—stereotypes that were probably at least partly based on some of the realities of that era, as depicted, for example, in *The Boys in the Band.* A lot of my fear was based on deep doubts about my own attractiveness and worth, and meeting someone like Lenny, who seemed to like me, was like a wonderful fantasy come true.

So how was this idyll shattered, and what did Buddhism have to do with it? Six months after becoming lovers, we found our own place—a fifth-floor walk-up—a hovel with the bathtub in the kitchen, in an ancient tenement on East 3rd Street on the Lower East Side of Manhattan. We immediately got involved with the burgeoning East Side "hippie" counterculture, in which being gay was accepted as either no big deal or a groovy defiance of straight society. We were both marking time in college, but LSD and other psychedelics were everywhere and proved much more engrossing than Latin or the English metaphysical poets. With psychedelics came the opening to a new world "beyond the doors of perception," a memorable phrase by poet William Blake. The experience might best be described as "mystic," an ineffable state, but one that recently has been well-characterized as "a hidden dimension of human consciousness in which the dichotomies of normal awareness are transcended in an intense experience of unity or communion with a hidden reality or presence."[2] I'd read about Zen, and had been very inspired by Jack Allen Kerouac's *Dharma Bums* and Ginsberg's Queer Buddhist-Hindu mystical rants when I was a teenager. With direct experience came an intense desire to find out more about this higher reality, and we started reading the few books then available, going from Timothy Leary's loopy psychedelic take on the *Tibetan Book of the Dead,* to Evans-Wentz's theosophical interpretation of the same book, to Alexandra David-Neel's exciting tales of flying lamas. By 1966 we had found our teacher, Geshe (Ngawang) Wangyal, a Kalmyk Mongol from the Crimean area of Russia, who had lived forty years in Tibet and was the first Tibetan Buddhist monk in America to teach Buddhism to Americans.

Geshe-la,[3] as we called him, was a most extraordinary person. His own teacher was the influential and mysterious Buriat Mongol lama Agvan Dorzhiev, a chief advisor to the Thirteenth Dalai Lama, and a key figure both in the revival of Buddhism among the Mongols in this century and the "great game" of Central Asian politics.[4] Geshe-la taught in the ordinary manner, reading and explaining texts to his students, but he taught even more powerfully in his everyday interactions, which could manifest themselves as immensely compassionate or exceedingly wrathful, which in all cases were meant to increase the student's awareness of her or his egocentricity and neuroses. In the apt words of one of his closest disciples, Jeffrey Hopkins, "He taught untiringly and was both the most beautiful and the most terrifying person I have known. To live with him was to live with emptiness."[5] Unlike the xenophobic Tibetans, Geshe-la was curious about other peoples and cultures and travelled extensively in China and India. He took a rare journey (for a lama at that time) to England in the 1930s with his student and friend, the gay English explorer, scholar, and musician Marco Pallis. Anticipating the Chinese suppression of Tibet, he emigrated to the United States in 1955 to minister to the Kalmyk community in New Jersey. He also taught Mongolian at Columbia University and began to teach Buddhism to American students, over the objections of Mongol traditionalists. As a man of great sagacity and practicality, he was a consummate "people-knower" and was well aware that a number of his students were gay, lesbian, or bisexual—a matter to which he seemed to assign no importance. He had enormous charisma, and his first teachings to Lenny and me, unlike the mystic secrets we had anticipated, were blunt injunctions to get away from drugs—especially LSD—find jobs, and show some compassion for our parents. Coming from him, these words were effective, as they would have been from nobody else. We saw him as the embodiment of Enlightenment.

Geshe-la always characterized spiritual development as "the maturation of people," or as he phrased it, to "ripen" (rhyming with "pippin"). Unfortunately, this process can't be rushed, so despite his influence, and my beginning to study Tibetan language and Buddhist practice, I was still a highly immature, insecure, self-centered kid. Lenny drudged away at a straight job at an uptown bank and was the principal financial support of our whole scene. We had moved "uptown" to 4th Street between Avenues A and B, a large apartment with a floating population of two to four friends who lived with us and various people crashing temporarily or just hanging out. Lenny would come home from work and find us listening to loud rock, jazz, Tibetan, or Indian music; talking foolishness; smoking hash; lounging around—all he wanted then was a little peace and privacy, but we just urged him to "cool out," get high, and teased him for being so uptight. Lenny didn't have the behavioral skills to assert himself then and just became more and more depressed and anxious. Finally, he fled to the monastery, as the only way out of an intolerable situation.

A couple of months without him brought me to my senses. I realized how unaware of his needs and how utterly insensitive I had been—this was a sobering insight, after I'd imagined, with the grandiosity of the young fueled by the hubris of that self-celebratory era, that I was a Bodhisattva, a Buddhist "saint," totally devoted to the needs of others! I visited him at the monastery a few times. I was further alarmed once by someone joking about how Lenny and one of the female students should get married, and I gave him assurances that things were going to change if he came back home.

He decided to do so. We were sitting with Geshe-la one evening, and he looked at us and said, "You two must stay together; you must help each other." We both agreed and have always considered that our true "wedding." We pledged our commitment in front of the person whom we considered a Buddha. It must have stuck, for twenty-seven years later we are still happily together, which seems a nearmiracle in these times.

By examining the attitude of traditional Buddhist cultures toward Queer people and same-sex friendship and sexuality and looking at Buddhist ways of relating to others, it is possible to see how Buddhism can be a positive part of other lesbigay couples' lives.

Throughout almost all of its history, in the many cultures in which it flourished, Buddhism has profoundly rejected what the benighted American political right calls "traditional family values." The basic paradigm is found in the life story of Sákyamuni, the Buddha (Awakened One). He was a very sheltered, upper-class young man, who was already married with a young son, when his first view of sick, aging, and dead people took away his pleasure in family life, and the sight of a homeless mendicant gave him hope of a way out. For Sákyamuni, no less than for the Jesus of the Gospels, the biological family was an impediment to spiritual growth, to be left behind if necessary. The very name for the traditional first step in serious Buddhist practice, entering the monastic state—literally means "leaving home." Friends have occasionally asked me about the "Buddhist marriage ceremony," and I have to tell them that this did not exist *per se* in traditional Buddhist societies, because marriage was not considered a religious occasion.* It was mainly with the development of modern forms of Buddhism influenced by Western (primarily Christian) models that specific marriage ceremonies have been created and enacted by Buddhist clerics.

The privileging of those who renounce social forms and obligations is not unique to Buddhism but has deep roots in Indian society. It is not difficult to understand the motivation for such renunciation, given the stiflingly hierarchical and rule-bound nature of the traditional Indian family, which requires the subordination of all individual needs to increase the prestige, wealth, and connections of the kin group. Women, especially, are treated as commodities, judged by the size of their dowries, future earning power, childbearing capacity, and other hard-eyed considerations. One can sense the joy of the early nun who wrote, "I'm free/free from kitchen drudgery/no longer a slave among my dirty cooking pots . . . and I'm through with my brutal husband . . . I purge lust with a sizzling

---

*Buddhist monks and nuns are not entirely removed from the laity, of course, and do perform some rituals relating to lay life, such as funerals or house-dedication ceremonies, but their role in marriages, if any, is rather peripheral. See Heinz Bechert and Richard Gombrich (Eds.). *The World of Buddhism: Buddhist Monks and Nuns in Society and Culture.* New York: Thames and Hudson, 1984, pp. 14, 188.

sound—POP/'O happiness,' meditate upon this as happiness."[6] But
the Indian renunciant is rarely a solitary figure; the Hindu *sadhus*
(wandering ascetics) are organized in distinct groups, and a noted
gay anthropologist with field experience in this area has asserted
that homosexual behavior is rather widespread among them. The
Buddhist monks and nuns were pledged to celibacy. Nevertheless,
they wandered in same-sex groups of brothers or sisters in the
Dharma (religious teaching), led by a preceptor (abbot or abbess)
who fulfilled the parental role. They had found a new family, with
rules to be sure, but whose objectives were to support each other's
spiritual development, having cut the attachments to wealth and lust
connected with the worldly family. Within a few hundred years,
most Buddhist renunciants were settled in monasteries or nunneries,
and the monastic community clearly functioned as a surrogate family, taking care of its members and inheriting their property at their
death. There seems at least an analogue here to the lesbian or gay
man who must often "leave home" to escape the abusive norms of
the heterosexual family and who then finds support from a chosen
family of Queer brothers and sisters who can nurture that person's
full human potential.[7]

Having grown up Queer in a Jewish working-class, "nonobser-
vant Orthodox" milieu, with its overpowering emphasis on marriage and family, Buddhism was the very breath of freedom for me.
Not only is reproductive heterosexuality not compulsory, it is not
even seen as particularly desirable, for anyone wanting to "wake
up" to reality and spiritual growth. *Homophobia is a nonissue in
Buddhism.* All sexual attachment is regarded as an unhealthy psychological factor because it is thought to lead to selfishness, anger,
envy, and other painful results. The gender or genders to which one
is attached is not of any significance. Buddhism has no sternly
parental creator-god to get angry at harmless human diversity. Consequently, Asian Buddhist societies have never seen the murderous
persecution of Queers that is found in the West. In Thailand, Sri
Lanka, Japan, and Tibet, same-sex sexual behavior was and is widespread, among laypeople and monastics, and nobody seems to
mind, as long as the layperson fulfills his or her obligation to marry
and produce children, and liaisons do not create too much of a

public scandal.* This acceptance may be part of the reason why so many lesbigays have found a congenial spiritual home in Buddhism, including well-known openly gay Buddhists such as Allen Ginsberg, John Giorno, and Issan Dorsey (a gay Zen abbot in San Francisco). It may also account for a number of lesbian and gay academics in Buddhist studies, as well as many lesbian and gay rank-and-file members of many American Buddhist centers, which, in my experience, have a significantly higher percentage of Queer folks than the general population.

In Asia, gender transgression was stigmatized, rather than same-sex sexuality *per se*. This was especially true regarding males who adopted the behavior, dress, and/or the receptive sexual activity "proper" to women. Such people were considered as a "third sex" in India from ancient times and were regarded as being disreputable and *déclassé*, although also at times as having special magical potency. They were generally ridiculed and devalued but accepted as part of society, like the female prostitutes with whom they were sometimes compared.[8] The Buddhist attitude toward this group was a negative one, clearly from the point of view of expedience. They were barred from becoming monks or nuns, mainly to protect the reputation of the monastic community. If the lay community, on whom monastics depended for their food and other necessities, came to see Buddhist monasteries as a hotbed of Queer sexuality, this would endanger the whole monastic order and its spiritual goals.[9]

Among monks and nuns, any penetrative sexual behavior was considered grounds for expulsion from the order. Nonpenetrative

---

*For example, in the Tibetan Buddhist cultural sphere, Owen Lattimore reported that Mongolian Buddhist monks justified same-sex sexuality on theological grounds; see his *Nomads and Commisars* (New York: Oxford University Press, 1962), p. 211. A young Japanese spy who lived disguised as a monk in Tibet also reported widespread homosexual behavior among lamas; see Hisao Kimura, *Japanese Agent in Tibet: My Ten Years of Travel in Disguise*, as told to Scott Berry (London: Serindia, 1990). Two modern prime ministers of Thailand have been widely known for their same-sex orientations, without damage to their political careers (Peter Jackson, personal communication, October 1995). For sympathetic tales of Japanese Buddhist monks and their love for young men see Ihara Saikaku, *The Great Mirror of Male Love*, translated by Paul G. Schalow (Stanford, CA: Stanford University Press, 1990).

acts were considered lesser and expiatable offenses, and one odd group of Tibetan monks—nonscholarly types who acted as police, security guards, musicians, and other important but low-status occupations—justified their notorious romances with handsome youths on the grounds that they practiced only intracrural intercourse.[10] Although same-sex relationships and sexual behavior were found in monasteries from China and Japan to Tibet, and were tolerated if not exploitative or too scandalous, they were nevertheless seen as falling short of the ideal of celibacy, distracting the monk or nun from the single-minded devotion to spiritual development and the welfare of others considered appropriate to renunciants.

In contrast to homosexual sex, same-sex friendship and companionship were highly valued in Buddhist culture. The popular literature of tales and fables, known to both laypeople and monastics, is consistent in its misogynist portrayal of wives and female lovers as lustful, unfaithful, and sinful, and its view of marriage as a sink of misery for both women and men. Friendship, on the other hand, is extolled in the highest terms, the model being the exemplary love and devotion of Buddha's closest attendant, Ānanda. Ānanda, whose name means "bliss" or "joy," is presented as having been the closest friend of the Buddha in many of their previous lives.[11] The ideal is that of the "virtuous friend" (*kalyāamitra*), who is motivated by the desire for the happiness and welfare, and especially the spiritual development, of his or her companion.

Ānanda is an intriguing figure, whose place in Buddhism could be seen as somewhat parallel to that of "John, the dearly beloved" in the Christian gospels—the Master's favorite disciple. So intense was Ānanda's affection for the Buddha that it was considered to have prevented him, despite his tremendous learning and piety, from achieving full liberation (arhatship) during the Buddha's lifetime. It was only after the latter's passing that Ānanda was able to free himself from all traces of the passions. His physical attractiveness was explicitly described, and he was popular among all the lay disciples, and especially among women. Ānanda is credited with persuading the Buddha to authorize the formation of a separate order of nuns, despite the Buddha's own qualms and the objections of other monks. According to traditional lore, Ānanda had personal reasons for his empathy with women. A tale describes one of his past lives as a blacksmith who committed adultery, for which he was punished in having to spend time in hell and subsequently undergoing fourteen human lives as a woman and a wife.[12] Not only does he appear to have a special sympathy for women and their concerns, but he also seems to have a connection to Queerness. One source cites a popular Thai belief that Ānanda had been born as a third-sex individual (*katheoy* in Thai) many times,[13] again as a result of sensual indulgence, and one of the canonical tales of his past lives represents him as having fallen in love with a handsome *nāga* (a type of serpent-deity) king, and pining away when the king no longer visited and embraced him.[14]

Although Buddhism may provide a comfortably nonhomophobic spiritual community, how is it specifically relevant to contemporary Queers and others, who are presented with the perennial problem, "How can we get along"? I believe the answer, or part of it, lies in the side of Buddhism that encourages prosocial attitudes. Starting with generating proper concern for one's own happiness and freedom from pain, one extends this feeling to one's parents, friends, and other benefactors, and eventually even to neutral and hostile people, cultivating joy in others' happiness and an impartial attitude.[15] This can help transform the initially selfish infatuation that we feel for people—wanting them all to ourselves, wanting to control them—into a true caring for and knowing the person as she or he is. These are the two kinds of love distinguished by Blake: the first "seeketh only Self to please/ To bind another to Its delight/Joys in another's' loss of ease/And builds a Hell in heaven's despite." The second, like the loving-kindness and compassion encouraged in Buddhism "seeketh not Itself to please/Nor for itself have any care/But for another gives its ease/And builds a Heaven in Hell's despair."[16]

Added to these social emotions is the basic Buddhist premise that the self is an ever-changing dynamic system, lacking any permanent core. The combination of this view with love and compassion is a way to synthesize seemingly diametric opposites—a warm, loving concern with detachment, which includes accepting the autonomy of others. This may seem like a tall order, but it certainly can be an ongoing ideal, given the attention and practice to sustain it. Such an attitude leads the way to true intimacy and a solution to the most common hassles I've seen in couples I've known personally, or worked with in couples therapy—alienating the other with criticism or control; the inability to hear each other; the fear of the other partner taking pleasure in friends or recreation that one doesn't like; and seeing the partner's changes or differences, the latter usually the very basis for the attraction, as a rejection of oneself. It has been the willingness to work at accepting each others' changes (I can never forget my initial horror at Lenny's first tattoo!), along with our supportive chosen family of gay and nongay friends, that has helped Lenny and me stay together and continue to evolve, and this seems a commonality in other successful relationships that I have encountered.

Although such attitudes obviously apply to any relationship, gays and lesbians may have some advantages in this process. The pride and self-acceptance that have come with gay liberation have broken down much self-hatred, fear, and rejection, and have enabled us to come together as a caring community, especially in response to the AIDS crisis. We can remember and use the pain of our oppression to increase empathy for others, and we are hopefully not bound by traditional heterosexual concepts of marriage, such as ownership and control. I think of a nongay friend, who recently confided that he hates going to large social gatherings, saying, "I have to go; my wife drags me to them." Middle-class heterosexual norms require couples to be together in social settings, under the penalty of shame and gossip. Queer couples seem more free to be individuals in relationships, rather than inseparable halves of a whole.

Buddhist practice has interacted with American culture and values to create new varieties of American Buddhism. This is inevitable because religions are always in the process of change, and the same kind of adaptation occurred when Buddhism encountered other already developed cultures, such as in China. How will American Buddhism deal with lesbian, bisexual, and gay Buddhists, and with gay Buddhist relationships, which are very different in form and content from anything known in traditional Asian societies? Some have already opted for assimilationist acceptance, similar to the liberal Christian or Jewish denominations that celebrate same-sex unions and welcome gays into their congregations. For example, the Soka Gakkai movement in America, an outgrowth of the Japanese Nichiren school, has approved marriage ceremonies for same-sex couples, the first Buddhist denomination to do so. Two representatives of Buddhist groups have testified in favor of same-sex marriage in Hawaii, and the Dalai Lama opined in a recent interview that gay relationships were fine, as long as the people involved "did not have any vows" (i.e., were not monks or nuns).

However, while the aforementioned are all beautiful and positive gestures, accepting loving, monogamous gay and lesbian couples is not much of a stretch for Buddhists, since there are no theological grounds not to do so. The challenge will be greater with the Queerer side of our community—the many nonexclusive relationships, probably the majority among gay male couples, group relationships, and S&M. The one clear rule in traditional Buddhist lay sexual morality is the prohibition of adultery, although even that doesn't formally apply to people who haven't taken special lay vows. Nonadulterous sexual play among ordinary laypeople is generally ignored.

However, this view of adultery is clearly a "conventional," or nonabsolute and situational one, based on the realities found in premodern Asian societies, predicated on the culture of marital ownership. To stealthily have sex with someone else's partner was seen as akin to using his oxen or milking his cow without his permission. Whether this would apply in a more open model of relationships, in which people did not consider their lovers or partners as property, needs to be the object of discussion among both Buddhist ethicists and Queer Buddhists. Some have already taken up this question.[14]

A further question relates to monasticism. Although mainstream traditional Buddhism has considered the monastic life as nearly the *sine qua non* for the higher development of ethics, contemplation, and wisdom, American monks and nuns have been rather few in number, with fewer still who remain permanently in the monastic life. My impression is that a fair number of these American Buddhist monastics, unlike their Asian counterparts, have at least in part chosen the celibate life as a retreat from sexuality and its conflicts, often (but not always) from gay and lesbian sexuality. This is a phenomenon one of our friends has called "the saffron closet" immersion in Buddhism, as a layperson or a monastic, as a strategy to avoid confrontation with one's forbidden or feared sexual orientation. Such avoidance is contrary to the Buddhist values of insight and self-acceptance and is terribly damaging to the individual's ability to relate genuinely to others in the world. I've known some folks who have emerged from these saffron closets and managed to joyfully connect to others emotionally and sexually, while maintaining their Buddhist identity and practice. The Hartford Street Zen Center in San Francisco, which maintains a hospice for people with AIDS, is one example of people living a Buddhist life openly as lesbians and gays. I hope that American Buddhism will continue to find such ways to provide affirming spaces for gays, lesbians, and bisexuals to develop as individuals and in multiple kinds of relationships, as part of a loving spiritual community.

NOTES

1. See Wayne Koestenbaum, *The Queen's Throat* (New York: Vintage Books, 1993), for a dishy account of what the opera line meant to young gay men in the 1950s and 1960s.

2. Jeffrey Kripal. *Kali's Child: The Mystical and the Erotic in the Life and Teachings of Ramakrishna.* Chicago: University of Chicago Press, 1995, p. 20.

3. *Geshe* is the Tibetan doctor of divinity degree; *la* is a Tibetan suffix denoting respect and affection.

4. For the fullest, though still inadequate, account of Dorzhiev's life, see John Snelling's *Buddhism in Russia* (Rockport, MA: Element, 1993).

5. Quoted in *Snow Lion Newsletter and Catalog*, Fall 1994, p. 29.

6. Translated by Anne Waldman and Andrew Schelling. "Songs of the Elders: From the Buddha's First Disciples." *Tricycle,* 5(2), Winter, 1995, p. 48.

7. See, for example, life stories in John Preston's *Hometowns: Gay Men Write About Where They Belong* (New York: Dutton, 1991), and the book he edited with Michael Lowenthal, *Friends and Lovers: Gay Men Write About Families They Create* (New York: Dutton, 1995).

8. For detailed information on queer identities in classical India, see Michael Sweet and Leonard Zwilling's "The First Medicalization: The Taxonomy and Etiology of Queerness in Classical Indian Medicine," *Journal of the History of Sexuality,* 3(1993): 590–607, and Leonard Zwilling and Michael Sweet, "'Like a City Ablaze': The Third Sex and the Creation of Sexuality in Jain Religious Literature," *Journal of the History of Sexuality,* 6(1996): 359–384. For the best study to date of the contemporary Indian transgender/third sex group, the *hijras,* see Serena Nanda, *Neither Man Nor Woman: The Hijras of India* (Belmont, CA: Wordsworth, 1990).

9. On the explanations given for this in the monastic literature, see Leonard Zwilling, "Homosexuality as Seen in Indian Buddhist Texts," in José Cabezón

(ed.), *Buddhism, Sexuality, and Gender* (Albany, NY: State University of New York Press, 1993).

10. On this group, the Dop-Dop (*Idab Idob*), who were found in the vast monastic universities of Central Tibet, see Melvyn C. Goldstein, "Study of the Ldad-Ldob," *Central Asian Journal, 9*(1964): 123–141.

11. This subject is excellently treated in John Garrett Jones, *Tales and Teachings of the Buddha* (London: George Allen & Unwin, 1979), especially pp. 105–116.

12. This story is found in the commentary to the *Dhammapada*, translated and edited by Eugene W. Burlingame, *Buddhist Legends*, Harvard Oriental Series, vols. 28–30. Cambridge: Harvard University Press, 1921; vol. 29, p. 25.

13. See Peter Jackson, "From *Kamma* to Unnatural Vice: Thai Buddhist Accounts of Homosexuality and AIDS," presented to the International Thai Studies Conference, London, 1993.

14. This is found in the Pali Jātakas, no. 253, *Maidaajātaka*, Fausböll, pp. 282–286.

15. This practice is described in detail in many popular books on Buddhist practice. See for example Geshe Kelsang Gyatso, *Universal Compassion* (London: Tharpa Publications, 1988), and Pema Chödrön, *Start Where You Are: A Guide to Compassionate Living* (Boston: Shambhala, 1994). For a psychotherapeutic application of these attitudes, see Michael Sweet and Craig G. Johnson, "Enhancing Empathy: The Interpersonal Implications of a Buddhist Meditation Technique," *Psychotherapy, 27*(1990): pp. 19–29.

16. From "The Clod and the Pebble," in his *Songs of Experience.*

17. For example, Robert Aitkin, a prominent nongay Zen Buddhist abbot and activist, stated in his testimony to the Hawaii Commission on Sexual Orientation and the Law on October 11, 1995, his view that the Buddhist precept of not engaging in sexual misconduct, usually taken to apply to adultery, means that "self-centered sexual conduct is inappropriate . . . Self-centered sex is exploitive sex, non-consensual sex, sex that harms others." (Taken from a reprint of his testimony posted on the Internet, from khush@flux.mindspring.com, January 6, 1996.)

Chapter 10

"With This Ring You Are Made Holy unto Me According to the Laws of Moses"
Celebrating and Sanctifying Lesbian and Gay Relationships and Families

Susan Talve

At the very first P-FLAG meeting I spoke at, a woman stood when I was done and said, "Had you been my son's rabbi, he might not have killed himself." I knew then, as I know now, that I can be part of this healing, but that it is much bigger than any one of us alone. The whole idea of celebrating and sanctifying must be in a community where people are willing to create models that may defy the popular culture but are better suited for the way we really want the world to be.

At the end of the service, we were all singing and whirling. While I held my infant son close, and wrapped him in the folds of my prayer shawl, the community of women that gathered each year for this retreat danced around us, celebrating the hope of a new generation, receiving blessings for ourselves by blessing him. One woman's eyes filled with tears. I knew that she and her partner had decided not to have a child of their own until their families and their communities welcomed that child with unconditional love. I handed her my son for a blessing, and I vowed to dedicate my ministry to creating a community that would celebrate her family and sanctify her relationships.

A few years later, always remembering my promise, I had the privilege of being part of forming a new congregation. Built into the principles was the vision of the founders to be inclusive. One of our first educational forums was a joint program with our local New

Jewish Agenda group to speak openly about the gay and lesbian Jewish experience. What we learned was that the few gay, lesbian, and bisexual Jews who maintained any kind of affiliation with the Jewish community at all "checked" their identities at the door. They neither felt safe nor welcomed with their partners. Many felt that their jobs would be at risk, being open in the congregation when they weren't "out" at work. They felt they were suspect if they came alone, and some even felt afraid for the custody of their children. Many people came to the forum, and once again I vowed to be part of a community that would celebrate gay and lesbian families and find ways to bless their relationships. But this time I was not making the promise alone. When our local Jewish newspaper covered the forum with an article that told the painful stories of our speakers, I was attacked for encouraging anti-Jewish lifestyles, "sin and abomination." The board of our new congregation responded with full support for me and an invitation to the gay and lesbian Jews of our city to know that there are people who care that they have been excluded. We committed ourselves to finding ways to create a safe space where we could all celebrate together, a space where we could say *kaddish* (the prayer for those who have died) together, and a space in which we could learn together. Over the past ten years, the work involved in creating this space has been both heartbreaking and rewarding, and the results both miraculous and imperfect.

We found that the first steps were internal. Because we had so few gay and lesbian members (people came to the synagogue but didn't join), the discussions at the board level about how to be inclusive always fell to asking, "Well, what do *they* want?" We knew that we had to overcome the "otherness" beneath the question. To have a healthy community, we had to search for the barriers both spiritual and physical that said to anyone not part of the perceived mainstream that they should "check" what made them different at the door. The inside barriers were our fears. We had fears about being labeled the "gay" congregation. We had fears about how this might influence or confuse the identities of our children, and we were afraid of AIDS. Just as we had built in strategies to overcome sexism, we began to build in strategies to overcome homophobia. Just as the equal inclusion of women in the synagogue made the experience more healthy and whole for everyone, we began to see how letting go of our homophobia was good for all of our souls and could even save the lives of the children we so wanted to protect.

Our goal was to create a community that would be open and safe. We made sure that every liturgy, ritual, and program was inclusive in form, language, and content. All the language we used and the stories we told included the presence of "partners" as well as "spouses" and "families" with a "parent" or "two parents," rather than assuming there would be mothers and fathers. Whenever we could, we used the biblical images of David and Jonathan, Ruth and Naomi, and the reconciliations of Jacob and Esau, Rachel and Leah, and others to help us to celebrate all healthy relationships without defining and limiting them.

I prayed for role models to emerge—members of the gay and lesbian Jewish community who would sit on the board, hold each other and their children in services, and teach our children in our school. A gay man with AIDS opened our hearts. He wanted to go to the *mikvah* (the Jewish ritual bath) before he died. The keepers of the *mikvah* would not permit it, though we had letters from many authorities that promised that he posed no threat to anyone's health. A family in the congregation emptied their hot tub and invited everyone to collect the rainwater that was needed to fill it in the prescribed way. We filled the hot tub with the living water that made it a sacred place, and he had his holy immersion. We knew that he had been a victim of both fear of AIDS and homophobia, but he helped us learn that we could stand together and make a difference for him and for ourselves.

Another gay man with AIDS began to worship with us. Before long, we were openly praying for his healing, and he was teaching in our school. When he could no longer care for himself, a sacred circle of close friends became his family. They cared for him in a way that his biological family could not and would not. They never left him alone, and he died in their loving arms. When it came time to bury him, it was clear who the mourners were. Yet, it still took a conscious leap to ascribe to his friends the status usually reserved for immediate family. Then, the community cared for his mourners, offering them comfort for their loss, honoring the mourners ribbons that they wore for him and recognizing the depth of their ongoing grief. When we say his name, we connect it with his sacred circle in the same way we connect all immediate family members to each other. We learned, once again, the precious lesson of celebrating and sanctifying gay and lesbian relationships.

As more role models were willing to share their lives openly, others began to join. A young man who spoke at our third High Holy Day Services said, "I am proud and gay and Jewish. In this world, no small miracle. Listen, and we will learn from each other how to bring about a society that will accept and respect us all. Again, no small miracle." A lesbian mother joined with her daughter. Also among those who joined were two women who had been partners for thirteen years, one of whom had been told by the rabbi of the congregation in which she grew up that it was best if she moved away from them so they would not be uncomfortable or embarrassed. At another service she said, "I am hopeful for the first time of finding a Jewish community in which to grow and celebrate all of me."

When there were enough members for the issues to be clearly "ours," the *Chavurah*, a fellowship or study group, was born. After six years of planning, five people met for a *Shabbat* (Sabbath) dinner in a member's home. Five years later, the Chavurah has a membership of well over 50 people who meet monthly to celebrate the Sabbath, learn together, and offer support to each other. The Chavurah has also become a precious resource for the congregation. The members represent the Jewish community and our congregation in many political and communal groups working for the healing of the larger community such as the Privacy Rights Education Project; Food Outreach (to provide meals for AIDS patients); Parents, Families, and Friends of Lesbians and Gays (P-FLAG); and Effort for AIDS, to name a few. Members of the Chavurah have led groups, taught adults and children, and provided meals and housing for our youth groups when they host conclaves. The Chavurah volunteered to host the *kiddush* (blessed food) for the Bat Mitzvah service of a young woman whose extended family lived out of town, once again expanding and enriching our definitions of family. Members of the Chavurah designed a program where they tell their stories to junior-high and high-school students in religious schools to end stereotypes and provide role models for young people finding their own voices and identities. The list goes on and on and is important because for each event, more connections are made among people building community together. In this context of more understanding and less ignorance, more love and less fear, gay and lesbian members are finding more opportunities to celebrate and sanctify their relationships, not just in quiet, secret corners, but in the heart of a vibrant and active congregation.

A while ago I officiated at the traditional wedding of a young couple meant to be together. The bride wore a full white wedding dress, there was a procession and attendants, and everyone was happy and grateful for the "normalcy" of it all. During the ceremony, I watched the bride's brother cry. "I'm always the emotional one," he said to me later. We both knew that there was more. I knew that he longed for what his sister had, a traditional wedding, the complete adoration and support of his parents and the promise of a loving family of his own. Without speaking, we hugged and wondered if he, as a gay man, could ever see his dreams come to be.

Jewish tradition teaches that the union of two separate souls in marriage is as great a miracle as the parting of the sea in the story of our exodus from Egypt. The preparation before, and the ritual, itself, are meant to lead the couple to *Kiddushin,* which means *holiness* and refers to the part of the ceremony where the two become one family. This transformation allows the couple to establish a *Shalom Bayit,* a house of peace, and from that holy place, peace spreads forth for the sake of the couple and for *tikkun,* the repair of the world.

I have known both gay and lesbian couples who have achieved this goal through many experiences and many years together. They have overcome both legal and social discrimination and have truly become family with each other without ritually making a commitment. I also know that many of these couples are reluctant to put themselves in the arms of their religious traditions and rituals comes from a lifetime of hurt caused by exclusion and judgment. For some, there is also an internalized, self-directed homophobia that lives in denial of the rights all human beings have to celebrate and sanctify the precious few sacred relationships we are privileged to have in a lifetime. Ashamed of who they are, they would never celebrate, even privately, anything concerning their relationships. Others are seeking new models for relationships outside of the ones presented as normative by heterosexual marriage. They blame unrealistic expectations and sexist role determinations for the high divorce rates and dissatisfaction they see in traditional marriages.

What felt most unjust was the lack of choice for gay and lesbian couples. I began to hear from some couples that wanted to participate in the more traditional models of marriage, believing that the preparations and sacred rituals would strengthen their commitment to their new family, demonstrate the support of their extended families, and increase their chances of building relationships that would last.

I began to meet with more and more gay and lesbian couples who wanted some kind of marriage ceremony for themselves. I found that whether the marriage ceremonies are quiet and private ones or extravagant galas, it seems essential to use the traditional words and rituals. It is also important to require that the couple commit to a divorce ritual if the marriage fails. Then, standing under the traditional wedding canopy as couples have done for generations, they recite the ancient words that accompany the exchange of rings: "With this ring you are made holy unto me according to the laws of Moses and the traditions of Israel." We say these words, recognizing the reach that they require the tradition to make. We say these words, knowing that using them to sanctify gay and lesbian marriage defies many generations of people who have died defending this tradition. And we say them, believing with all our hearts that these words and ancient traditions do work to help transform couples into families and that each new family will create one more *Shalom Bayit,* one more peaceful place that not only will transform these lives but also will make the whole world a more peaceful place because of them. Because of this belief, it is a holy task to work to change the laws of our states to make gay and lesbian marriages legal as well.

In all of our experiences, the common theme has been that to celebrate and sanctify gay and lesbian relationships there have to be safe and loving places for gay, lesbian, and bisexual human beings to sanctify and celebrate all the sacred moments and passages of their lives. At the very first P-FLAG meeting I spoke at, a woman stood when I was done and said, "Had you been my son's rabbi, he might not have killed himself." I knew then as I know now that I can be part of this healing, but that it is much bigger than any one of us alone. The whole idea of celebrating and sanctifying must be in a community where people are willing to create models that may defy the popular culture but are better suited for the way we really want the world to be.

I recently received a letter that gives me hope that if we do continue to create these new models that stretch the notions of family and relationships and make more possibilities to sanctify and celebrate the holy spaces and relationships between us, we will grow to be healthier and happier human beings, which will in turn help lead us to more peace and less suffering. After her seventeen-year-old son "came out" to her, a member of our congregation wrote the following:

> *What is most important to me is how my son feels about himself. Having grown up with so much shame in my life, I detest that he feel at all ashamed about his sexual preference. What I see is, he doesn't. He wishes that it were different sometimes, that he was [sic] heterosexual, but he has no feelings of "wrongness." As he and I talked about it (because I don't feel any shame either), what we both realized is that we have made our world up of people for whom being gay is "no big deal." The community to which we are both, in our own ways, strongly connected—our Jewish home—welcomes and honors gays and lesbians. It is no problem for my son to be Jewish and gay. He knows, he really knows, that his rabbi and his community love him, and he never has to pretend to be someone else, worry about keeping any secrets, or feel any shame. Neither do I. We are truly blessed.*

It seems that we human beings have a long way to go to figure out how to live together more peacefully. I'm sure that as the Ba'al Shem Tov[1] said, as human beings that are destined to be together find each other, and we are able to sanctify the new families that they form, their streams of light will flow together, and a single united light will go forth from their united beings, leading all of us to a time and place that is more peaceful and a true celebration of all creation.

NOTE

1. Rabbi Israel ben Eliezer, founder of Hasidism.

Chapter 11

A Family Friend
Paul's Letter to the Romans as a Source of Affirmation for Queers and Their Families

Thomas Hanks

When we inquire about what kind of communities Paul sought to encourage and empower with his greetings in Romans 16, the following three types stand out: feminist/womanist, poor, and gender-bender.

In 1989, my apartment in Buenos Aires was jammed with exuberant Argentines, smiling often through their tears as Metropolitan Community Church (MCC) pastor Roberto Gonzalez conducted what we believe to be the first gay marriage in the country (actually a blessing, with an exchange of promises). Then in July 1995, as we gathered in Rio de Janeiro, Brazil for the International Lesbian and Gay Association (ILGA) conference, a lesbian couple contacted me, requesting a similar service for their relationship. Again, Roberto was present and agreed to do the service—but news spread and soon some thirty gay and lesbian couples were turning the event into the first "mass wedding" for same-sex couples in Latin America. Roberto managed to get faxed from the Metropolitan Community Church Los Angeles headquarters the English liturgy that Troy Perry had used for the massive blessing during the March on Washington in 1993, which we barely managed to get translated and adapted in time. The press got wind of the event, sending many of the closeted participants to the "back pews" in the hotel meeting room.

For many who only read about such services in the press, they sound weird and alienating. Surely there must be a lot in the Bible against such services and in support of the traditional family, they

think. Pulpits and media journalists continually support such
claims.

Despite the incredible ideological hype from both political and
religious propaganda machines, the Bible never refers to "the family." Biblical traditionalists who stick with the sixteenth-century
King James Version will be closer to the truth, since the older, more
literal translations say such things as: "Believe on the Lord Jesus
Christ, and thou shalt be saved and thy *house*" (Acts 16:31). *House*
is inaccurately translated as "family" in most modern versions, or
the occasionally helpful, "household."

In the older, more literal, translations, other common mainstays
of modern mistranslations of the Bible also are totally absent. We
find neither reference to homosexuals (or heterosexuals, bisexuals,
or even sex!), nor to ethics or morals. The Bible, in fact, in its
original languages of Hebrew and Greek, consistently refers to the
"house/household" commonly involving everyone living under the
same roof or on the same patriarchal turf (earlier in tents).

Biblical scholar L. William Countryman conveniently summa-
rizes extensive data long familiar to New Testament students, dem-
onstrating Jesus's strong critique of the idolatry that permits devotion to household members to usurp loyalty to God and love for
one's neighbor.[1] According to Luke's Gospel, Jesus even went so
far as to commend his own lifestyle as an itinerant prophet: "If
anyone comes to me and does not hate his own father and mother
and wife and children and brothers and sisters, yes, and even his
own life, he cannot be my disciple" (Luke 14:26). Whatever con-
trasts we may find between Jesus's teaching and that of Paul, Countryman points out the basic continuity in Paul's option for the lifestyle of an unmarried, impoverished, itinerant prophet.[2] Of the
other New Testament authors, only Peter and Jude were married,
and the New Testament commonly envisions the house churches as
taking the place of patriarchal households in the divine program.[3]

In a culture of increasing biblical illiteracy, the Bible serves
principally as an oppressive icon. It may seem like an exercise in
futility to try to point out that a close reading of the Bible actually
subverts and deconstructs the common idolatry of the modern
nuclear family.[4] Paul's letter to the Romans, which has been cited
from monarchists to Nazis to demand obedience to violent autho-

ritarian regimes (13:1–7) and by homophobes to promote violence against gay men and lesbians (1:26–27), would seem to be the last place we might expect to look for a subversive deconstruction of modern family idolatry. However, Paul's liberationist credentials suffer most from the popular tendency to cite texts out of context for ideological purposes, neglecting to read the letter from start to finish or from finish to start, which modern readers may often find a more helpful approach.

Recent studies of Paul's letter to the Romans demonstrate that, contrary to traditional readings, Paul's main point does not become clear until the end of the letter. Traditional efforts to isolate Paul's earlier points about universal human sinfulness (Romans 3) or justification by faith alone (Romans 4) fail to take into account Paul's missionary context and purpose. The five subversive house churches that had sprung up in Rome under Nero's nose tended to split between two factions: Jews who had acknowledged Jesus as their messiah, and gentile believers ingrafted ("contrary to nature," the same word used in Romans 1) into the olive tree of Judaism (Romans 11). As an itinerant prophet and missionary, Paul aimed to visit Rome and then use the five house churches as a support basis for reaching Spain; hence, his eagerness that the house churches not split into warring factions over controverted aspects of the gentile lifestyle, which Jews found incompatible with the Torah and tradition. In regard to this he writes, "Accept one another just as Christ accepted you (both Jews and gentiles), in order to bring praise to God" (15:6).

In Chapter 16, then, Paul greets people he knew personally in the five house churches, revealing in greater depth his vision for communities that would represent God's liberating project for all of humanity. While God's purposes in the house churches included justice, love, and wisdom, foundational to these virtues was liberation and authentic freedom (8:21). In his earlier letter to the Galatians, freedom also was made fundamental (5:1,13), and Paul warned that certain false brothers "infiltrated our ranks to spy out the freedom we have in Christ Jesus" (2:4). In an age when "church" calls forth images of St. Peter's in Rome or St. Patrick's in New York, with all their associations of tyranny, bigotry, and oppression, it is difficult for us to imagine the original historical context of Paul's writing when house churches were subversive focal points of shocking freedom (unparalleled and unrivaled in the ancient world) and not bulwarks of complacent bourgeois conformity. Can anyone imagine someone today sneaking into the typical suburban church to spy out examples of subversive freedom? In Eastern Europe, however, before the collapse of the Soviet Empire, Protestant churches commonly offered the only safe space for gay men and lesbians to meet. When we inquire as to what kind of communities Paul sought to encourage and empower with his greetings in Romans 16, three types stand out: feminist/womanist, poor, and gender-bender.

Male commentators and preachers have long neglected the feminist/womanist perspective. Romans 16 has become a major focus of modern feminist and womanist scholarship because of the emphasis on women leaders evident in the chapter. In his commendation of the Reverend Phoebe, Romans 1:1–2, Paul designates her a minister/deacon of her church in Cenchrea (near Corinth in Greece). She had been a patroness of many, including Paul himself. Phoebe probably had to visit Rome for legal business (likely to defend from male predators her inherited property), and so was entrusted with Paul's letter to the five house churches in Rome. Soon the letter Phoebe faithfully delivered stood at the head of the churches' collection of Pauline correspondence as the longest and most profound exposition of the Apostle's message.*

With regard to Paul's greeting of Prisca and Aquila (1:3–4), Prisca/Priscilla is usually named first in the New Testament. Prisca was one of the first church leaders to preach the Gospel in Rome. It may well have been her controversial proclamation that touched off

---

*In 386 C.E., Augustine picked up the letter, read Romans 13:11–14 and was converted. From 1515–1516, Martin Luther expounded Romans in the light of the Psalms' teaching on faith as trust, thus rediscovered Paul's radical teaching about justification by faith alone, and sparked the Protestant Reformation. In 1738, John Wesley listened to Moravian brethren read Luther's preface to Romans, and felt his heart "strangely warmed." Soon the Methodist revival broke out in England. In 1919, Swiss theologian Karl Barth's commentary fell "like a bomb on the playground of the theologians" in postwar Europe. Such illustrations from church history (male written) force us to ask how different history might have been had Phoebe lost the letter Paul entrusted to her!

riots, resulting in the Emperor Claudius's edict (49 C.E.) expelling all "Jews" from Rome, including those who acknowledged Jesus as the Messiah. Prisca and Aquila first became political exiles in Corinth. They later settled in Ephesus, where Prisca proceeded to correct the theology of the learned and eloquent Apollos (Acts 18:26). After the death of Claudius, Prisca and Aquila were able to return to Rome (55–56 C.E.). Apollos may have later written the epistle to the Hebrews to the house churches there, when Prisca was still a "leader" (65–66 C.E.; cf. Heb. 13:7, 17, 24). Prisca displayed the "manly" virtue of courage (Rom. 16:4; cf. 1 Cor. 16:13, literally "play the man"), risking her life for Paul. Thus Paul singles out a female church leader as the first to receive his greeting. As fellow tent makers, Prisca and Aquila were probably chosen as his forerunners and emissaries to the house churches in Romans 1:3.

In Romans 13:7, Paul refers to a married couple, Andronicus and his wife Junia, and designates each with the highest New Testament title of "apostle." That Junia was a woman and an apostle was commonly acknowledged throughout the patristic period, but medieval scribes changed her name to a masculine form to censure this fact.

In the commendation (Rom. 16:1–2) and fifteen greetings (16:3–16) Paul refers to twenty-nine persons—ten women and nineteen men. Only three of the nineteen men are designated church leaders, while seven of the ten women are specifically commended for their leadership in the church (1–2, 3–5a,6a,7a,12). From the available evidence, modern scholars conclude that the five Roman house churches were founded and led mainly by charismatically gifted women. Schmithals points out that this leadership pattern, dependent on charismatic gifts, was characteristic of the more Hellenistic churches, while the patriarchal pattern of exclusive male elders (presbyters) prevailed in more judaistic churches.[5]

Paul addresses the poor, oppressed, and marginalized. Because some two-thirds of the persons Paul dignifies with a personal greeting bore names common to the slave class (ten of twenty-four, plus the slaves in the two households mentioned in 16:10–11), modern scholars conclude that the members of the early Roman house churches came predominantly from the lower social strata. Jews in Rome were marginalized and common objects of persecution, and six of the twenty-four persons Paul mentions were apparently Jewish. Concern for the poor also may be reflected in Phoebe's office of deacon (in Cenchrea) and in the collection Paul proposed to carry to Jerusalem for the poor saints there (15:25–27, 31). Although not as explicit as Jesus (Luke 4:18–19), Paul clearly identified himself with poor "debtors" (Rom. 16:16–17), sought to proclaim "good news to the poor," and established house churches that would embody solidarity with the poor (see also 1 Cor. 11:17–22).

Finally, Paul speaks to the gender-benders. Suburban churches commonly attract and give priority to the modern ideal nuclear family (a married couple with 2.2 children). Hence, for contemporary readers, perhaps the most shocking aspect of Romans 16 is the predominance of the gender-bending "households" that the apostle dignifies and empowers with his personal greeting. In a culture where greetings were of great social importance, Paul addresses with approval and supports a veritable sociological "zoo" of domestic arrangements!

Of the twenty-four persons greeted, we find that only six are married and that none of the three couples represents a typical patriarchal household: Prisca is presented as the dominant partner (3–4); the apostle Junia has an egalitarian marriage with her apostle husband; and in the case of the remaining couple, it is the male gender-bender who bears the name *Philologus* (meaning "talkative"—supposedly a feminine trait!)[6] Thus, even the six married persons are all gender-benders of sorts, showing the diversity of marriage arrangements possible in the early churches.

The remaining eighteen persons greeted are unmarried, and the gender-bending produces some astonishing pretzels of nonconformity to standard patriarchal expectations! Of the fifteen single men greeted, Paul greets three simply because they are "beloved" by him—a purely emotional bond (Rom. 16:5, 8–9). We may include Phoebe plus the six women greeted because they are church leaders and co-workers with the apostle. Only one woman is designated by Paul as "beloved," but in her case she is also called a co-worker (16:6, 12b). Three men and two women (16:6, 12b) are greeted simply as individuals with no indication of their household or domestic situation.

In the households of gender-benders whom Paul dignifies and supports with special greetings we have the following people:

- Two unmarried men living together (16:8; Urbanaus is a "co-worker," while Stachys is a "beloved," so they manage to complement each other in a same-sex living arrangement).
- Paul's "co-workers" Tryphaena and Tryphosa (16:12), probably sisters like Mary and Martha.
- Rufus (the "redhead"), a (confirmed?) bachelor living with his mother (16:13).
- A household consisting of five single men who live with unnumbered Christian "brothers" (probably their slaves and servants; 16:4).
- Philologus and his wife (16:15), who live with bachelor Nereus, his sister, and another single man (Olympas).
- Unnamed Christian slaves who live in two households headed by unconverted men (16:10–11).

Of the twenty-four persons greeted, only Philologus and his wife even approximate the modern type of nuclear family idealized by church and society. Undoubtedly Philologus had plenty to talk about with his wife, surrounded as they were by such a shocking variety of early Christian households! Yet instead of seeking to marginalize, criticize, and destroy the self-esteem of this "motly" collection, Paul seeks to dignify and empower all of his beloved friends and diligent co-workers, whatever their domestic arrangements, with a special personal word of greeting. Priority is even given to the more nonconformist representatives, with talkative Philologus and his long-suffering wife placed near the end of the list.

Paul's final touch in this shocking list of greetings is to command everyone to kiss each other (16:16; cf. 1 Cor. 16:20; 2 Cor. 13:21; 1 Thes. 5:26; 1 Pet. 5:14). The apostolic command that involved males publicly kissing each other is the standard greeting in Buenos Aires (as I discovered to my great discomfort when I moved there from Costa Rica), but it is illegal on the streets of homophobic London and many other places. I often wonder what would happen if a male in Jerry Falwell's church tried to greet Jerry with a kiss (in obedience to Paul's and Peter's repeated, clear commands) after one of his bigoted homophobic diatribes that pass for sermons.

The picture is completed in Romans 16:21–24, where Paul includes greetings from Timothy and seven other single men, apparently all housed together under the roof of their host Gaius. German New Testament scholar Gerd Theissen cites extensive evidence and studies concluding that Paul was a repressed homosexual, a conclusion almost universally ignored in scholarly circles, although never refuted.[7] Romans, read to the end, may represent Paul's spiritual and emotional pilgrimage from a rhetorical use of common Jewish homophobia (1:24–27, where, as Countryman has shown, same-sex activities are categorized as "unclean," but not explicitly sinful), to the revolutionary, liberating insights that now "all things are clean" (14:20) and that God delights to act "contrary to nature" (11:24). Probably Paul's sexual orientation and practice, and the interpretation of Romans, will remain items of sharp debate for the foreseeable future. However, what is undeniable is that Paul's gender-bending lifestyle was such that he would not be permitted to rent an apartment in many residential areas in the United States. And he, accompanied by Timothy or alone, would never be permitted to light an Advent candle, much less preach, in many suburban churches. The same should be said for the gender-benders and sexual minorities that constituted the overwhelming majority of the house churches in Rome centuries before there was a pope, a Saint Peter's basilica, and an institution perverted to serve the interests of the wealthy, especially males, and nuclear families.

Only by scrutinizing the diversity of the early house churches in Rome can we properly understand divisions and scandals (16:17–20). Today it is common to hear prosperous, married, male clergy attack anyone who seeks to subvert their privilege and authority. In this kind of "majority, integrative propaganda," the scandals and divisions that threaten the unity and purity of the church are always blamed on those Latin American liberation theologians who advocate an "option for the poor," or those pastoral voices who espouse ordination and church leadership for women and gender-benders.

When Paul evidently snatches the pen from the hand of his secretary-scribe Tertius and proceeds to denounce those who create divisions and scandals (16:17–20), he obviously identifies the problem elsewhere. Anyone who does not follow Jesus in his special com-

mitment to the poor, his affirming of women in leadership, in digni-
fying gender-benders and sexual minorities are the ones who create
divisions and scandals. It is precisely the affluent, white, married,
male clergy who use their education and eloquence ("fair and flat-
tering words") to serve their own appetites for power and privilege.
Paul says "watch out" for those types and don't follow them; turn
away from them. These self-appointed "leaders" will stop being
leaders only when the rest of us stop following them!

Paul's letter to the Romans eventually became a mighty standard
in the defense of what the Catholic Church considered "orthodox"
teaching; hence, the tremendous irony of the final doxology
(16:25–27), which did not form part of the earliest Greek manu-
scripts. But where did it come from? In the second century C.E., the
theologians who considered themselves "orthodox" faced the first
major Christian heretic, Marcion. Many churches followed the
teaching of Marcion, and when they circulated a somewhat reduced
version of Romans, they composed the beautiful doxology that now
concludes the letter (cf. the conclusion to the Lord's Prayer).
Romans thus bears witness that God can speak to the church even
through liturgies from heretics.[8]

Recent scholarly study of Paul's letter to the Romans leaves
fundamental questions unanswered, and stranger ones remain
unasked. For example, gender studies, which have become virtually
passé in other disciplines, seem to be systematically avoided, even
though the major study on Pauline psychology pointed out more
than a decade ago that Paul probably was a repressed homosexual.[9]
While no book has been dissected with such care, the question of
the way Paul's sexual orientation affected the development of his
letter to the Romans has been left untouched. Whereas women and
people of color play an increasingly prominent role in other academic areas, it is shocking and perplexing to walk into the Society
of Biblical Literature seminar on Paul in recent years and see a
room of some 100 white men, with perhaps two women and one
person of color. Is this Paul's fault, or the Christian churches' fault
(for using his writings to support slavery and oppose misogyny)? Is
society correct in perceiving in Paul an apostle of oppression
instead of an apostle of liberation? Or has the academy so limited
the questions and methodology as to render Paul irrelevant in the

struggle for human freedom? Although influential Latin American theologians have made important contributions to Pauline studies, their works, questions, and conclusions are systematically ignored. Academic study of Paul seems well on its way to becoming a sterile debate between uptight British and American scholars who seem afraid to raise questions about Paul's sexuality and the use and abuse of his teaching in church and society today. Outside the academic forum, of course, several participants have revealed their homophobia (Richard Hays, James D. G. Dunn), while others have made persistent and valiant attempts to see sexual minorities included in society and the church without discrimination (Robin Scroggs, Victor Furnish, George Edwards).

Some current directions in Pauline studies offer some promise to Queers. For example, Douglas A. Campbell points out that in Romans 1–3, Paul sets forth much that does not actually represent his own position, including natural theology, and that commonly we err when "we characterize him in terms of his opponents' theology, a theology that he himself was deeply opposed to."[10] Following Countryman, Campbell might have raised the question whether this has not been done in the traditional interpretation of Romans 1:24–27, which sees Paul supporting the homophobia of his contemporary Jews, instead of setting it up for later refutation, but Campbell avoids this debate.

Marty L. Reid points out that in antiquity even standard works on rhetoric, such as Quintilian, noted that "the same word is used in two different meanings."[11] This could imply that Paul in fact makes no reference to lesbian sex, since "against nature" in Romans 1:26 need not mean the same thing as it does in 1:27. That would bring Romans into line with the other handful of biblical texts that say something about same-sex acts—they speak only of male acts and may only refer to such acts as are harmful to the neighbor (violence, abuse of minors, idolatrous prostitution; Romans 13:8–10).

Finally, Paul W. Meyer, citing Hays in part, says, "The resurrection does not eradicate the death of Jesus, but makes it an 'apocalyptic event,' and Paul uses apocalyptic categories and traditions to make clear what God's raising of this Jesus makes this event mean: 'the very structure of reality is changed.'"[12] However, if that most shameful act of being crucified may be so transformed by the resurrection, how much more (and this may be Paul's eventual point in Romans) can male same-sex acts be transformed in the light of the resurrection? Romans may thus be read as reflecting Paul's personal struggle to "come out" and accept his sexual orientation as God's gift. Otherwise why does he deconstruct all the points in what at first glance appears to be common Jewish homophobic diatribe in Romans 1:24–27?

A careful reading of Romans 16 reveals to us a Paul who avoided the either/or dichotomies typical of traditional patriarchal male thought. Inspired by God's spirit (verbally and inerrantly, some would insist), Paul could affirm and encourage with his personal greeting the three married couples known to him ("families" in the modern sense) without insulting and destroying the dignity of the majority in the five house churches, who found themselves in other domestic arrangements. In fact, in these urban house churches, where domestic arrangements typical of gender-benders and sexual minorities statistically were overwhelmingly predominant, Paul goes out of his way to make clear that those unmarried (like himself; Jesus; the apostles, except Peter; and Paul's closest collaborators) were in no way to be treated as second-class citizens.

Today, the churches that insist most on the inspiration, authority, and veracity of the Bible are those that have become most idolatrous with their "either/or" dichotomies that seek to support traditional nuclear families, while insulting, harming, and seeking to destroy all those who find themselves in other domestic arrangements. Nowhere is their bigotry, hypocrisy, and gross ignorance of actual biblical text made more clear. In the patriarchal cultures of biblical times, children were married off as soon as they were sexually mature. Patriarchal commands in the Bible to regulate procreation and property inheritance made considerable sense in that context, originally agrarian. However, today we have churches which make the Bible their icon but which would never dream of using the Bible to help deconstruct the modern invention of "adolescence," the ten-to-fifteen-year period of maximum male sexual drive, which churches address with non-biblical demands of sexual abstinence, in an age of rampant AIDS, with idiotic homilies against condoms. Professor Richard A. Posner, a conservative Reagan judicial appointee, cites statistics indicating that in the United States the cases of AIDS among Roman Catholic priests is now 27 *times* (not percent!) that of the population as a whole.[13] Yet Pope John Paul comes to America, blames his seminaries for accepting students for the purportedly celibate priesthood who are 70 percent homosexual, and then pleads for recruitment of more clergy like the revolution in Goya's famous painting devouring its own children.

At this writing (November 1995), Brazil, with its long history of sex-positive culture, seems poised to take the leadership in liberation for sexual minorities. More than 150 communities already have passed antidiscrimination laws to protect gays and lesbians, and this month the legislature is expected to pass a national law to the same effect. In the spring of 1996, the legislature is expected to pass the first "gay marriage" (civil union) law to come into effect outside of northern Europe.

In the coverage of the ILGA conference in Rio de Janeiro in July 1995, the Brazilian press distinguished itself for the breadth and depth of its coverage of the conference and related issues, and this affected press coverage in other Latin American nations, and even in the United States. John Doner and Pepe Hernandez, in their historic trip visiting each country in Latin America by bus in 1994, interviewed one gay couple in Brazil who has even managed to adopt a child (something not permitted by European laws to date).

From Paul's example in Romans 16, we see how leaders can be supportive of traditional families without becoming viciously destructive of the dignity and stability of other kinds of households. Paul's norm was simply the kind of neighbor-love that does not "harm" the neighbor (13:8–10), whether the neighbor was involved in a traditional marriage, was single, or sought comfort and stability in another kind of household. Paul's letter also is a prime example of how to think globally and act locally. Even our best leaders in the struggle for lesbigay liberation in the United States give the impression that we can move ahead on our own, have nothing to learn from other nations, and no responsibility to share our own insights and resources.

In the United States, and even more in Europe, I commonly encounter lesbigay leaders who recognize homophobic religions as the main ideological obstacle, but often, instead of informing themselves about these forces, they profess indifference and studied ignorance of religious phenomena; "religious allergies" would appear to be the major cause for political defeats. In Latin America, liberation theologies provide a powerful answer to homophobic religious forces.[14] Leading liberation theologians have been slow in applying their insights to the oppression of sexual minorities. Lesbigay leaders, however, have begun to make major use of liberationist insights, and even atheists and agnostics among them have learned how to refute decisively homophobic religious leaders in the media—encounters that are increasingly common. If lesbigay leaders in the First World begin to learn how to think globally as they seek to act locally, they will discover that Latin America has much more to give than it needs to receive.

NOTES

1. L. William Countryman. *Dirt Greed and Sex in the New Testament*. Philadelphia: Fortress, pp. 168–189.

2. Countryman, pp. 190–220.

3. Countryman, pp. 221–234.

4. Janet F. Fishburn. *Confronting the Idolatry of the Family: A New Vision for the Household of God*. Nashville: Abington Press, 1991.

5. Walter Schmithals. *Der Roemerbrief: Ein Kommentar*. Gutersloh, Germany: Mohn, 1988, p. 555

6. James D.G. Dunn. *Romans* (Word Bible Commentary 38a & b). Dallas: Word, 1988, p. 900.

7. Gerd Theissen. *Psychological Aspects of Pauline Theology*. Philadelphia: Fortress, 1987, p. 26.

8. Dunn, p. 913.

9. Theissen, p. 26.

10. Douglas A. Campbell. "A Rhetorical Suggestion Concerning Romans 2." Society of Biblical Literature 1995 Seminar Papers, ed. by Eugene H. Lovering Jr., Atlanta: Scholars Press, 1, p. 126.

11. Marty L. Reid. "Paul's Rhetoric of Mutuality: A Rhetorical Reading of Romans." Society of Biblical Literature, 1995, Seminar Papers, p. 126.

12. Paul W. Meyer. *Pauline Theology: Some Thoughts for a Pause for its Pursuit*. Society of Biblical Literature, 1995, Seminar Papers, p. 702.

13. Posner, Richard A. *1992 Sex and Reason*. Cambridge: Harvard University Press, 1992, p. 155.

14. Richard Cleaver. *Know My Name: A Gay Liberation Theology*. Louisville: Westminster John Knox, 1995.

Chapter 12

Dancing Bears, Performing Husbands, and the Tyranny of the Family

Eric Rofes

The family construct is often accompanied—even in its Queer versions—by a privileging of image over reality, longevity over functionality, conformity over liberation. As these assumptions and values, which constitute the foundations of even liberal reappropriations of "family," infiltrate all levels and configurations of human relationships, I want to step back and recalculate the gains and losses of this strategy and reconsider whether authenticity, integrity, and freedom can survive the dogged tyranny of the family.

A vast, persistent longing for family reverberates throughout the land. Although it appears most relentlessly in the work of champions of "traditional family values," the mass communal yearning for family also echoes throughout the rhetoric of liberals and progressives. We may tussle over the definition of "family," but all seem to share in the belief that some kind of family, be it a couple, with or without children; a network of friends; or a multigenerational household collective, must serve to anchor our lives. We see needs—social, spiritual, sexual—that we believe can only be met through family formations.

The rising Queer quest for recognition of "our families" has long made me uncomfortable, even before I could identify the sources of my concern. The representation of our couplings and communal forms as "families" has seemed misguided. The ascension of marriage rights to the top of the gay political agenda has filled me with misgivings. A ubiquitous demand for access to "our children" through battles over insemination, adoption, and custody rights has inspired inner conflict. Most of all, the unexamined and unabashed rhetorical embrace of "family" in Queer discourse has triggered my hypervigilance and long-standing concerns for the integrity of authentic gay male social formations.

We're living through times when the lesbian and gay press offers a range of evidence affirming this tidal wave of "profamily" sentiment among Queers. In 1995, you can open up your local gay newspaper and turn to a column headlined "Family Values Key to Gay Rights."[1] In Tulsa, Oklahoma, it would be possible—even likely—to mistake the local Queer paper at a newsstand for a Christian Right publication, because its masthead proclaims in capital letters the name of the paper: *Tulsa Family News*. At the same time, a national "therapy-related" magazine for "lesbians, gays, bisexuals, and their relations" has recently been launched under the name *In the Family*.[2] One paper reports a San Francisco lesbian organization kicking off its first "Family Day" celebration. An organizer told the media, "We're doing this because we know that it will be bringing really positive images of ourselves and our families to light."[3] Perhaps the most ironic "profamily" action I've seen reported in the gay press focused on a male couple who spent five years pursuing a lawsuit against the District of Columbia's refusal to grant them a marriage license. Only when the Court of Appeals refused their case did they acknowledge that they had split up over a year and a half earlier.[4]

I understand and support some of the reasons Queers seem to be wrapping themselves in the American flag and reappropriating the construct of family. Courts of law must be stopped from severing bonds between children and their Queer parents. Health care workers must be stopped from restricting Queers from their lovers' hospital rooms. Corporations and the state must be stopped from awarding an array of economic benefits to heterosexual couples only. Yet a failure to deeply scrutinize the values and theoretical underpinnings of contemporary family rhetoric allows for the transfer of a range of abuses of power, authority, and economic privilege from HetAmeriKa into the Queer nation. Quite separate from promoting constructs of childhood, which dominate through infantilization, right-wing and liberal veneration of the family fails to examine ways in which this unit serves as an economic building block of a repressive, patriarchal social order.

Although radical right pundits insist that strong families are the building blocks of strong communities, I believe an extreme and undue emphasis on the family unit has seriously undermined the ability to create and maintain authentic community in America.[5] *Under the guise of caring for our families, energy is channeled by narrow self-interest and bound up in an intensive and privatized experience of interpersonal dysfunction.* People carry the unmet needs and untreated wounds that have been gestating in their families of origin into organizational and community life. We fearfully ponder the increasing inability of our nation's citizenry to fully function within participatory democracy, without identifying the family as a mass boot camp, producing a culture of disempowered victims and victimizers. Instead of being a period when an emerging consensus demands the increasing democratization of family, the 1990s brings escalating attempts to conceptualize children as colonial subjects and to pack stadiums full of patriarchal Promise Keepers vowing to reassert their rightful place as head of the family unit.[6]

I do not consider myself a survivor of abuse in my family of origin. My white, Jewish, middle-class parents created a suburban family life with all of the functionality and dysfunctionality of the times. I also have not had difficulty forming and nurturing intimate bonds with others. My closest friends remain primarily people with whom I "came out" twenty years ago, and I am entering my seventh year of living with the same man. Many consider me deeply committed to forging and strengthening bonds of friendship, desire, and love among people of all genders and sexual identities. My critique of the family in general—and of the "gay family" in particular—does not arise out of frustrations and failings in my own life.

Instead, my dissatisfaction with the increasingly relentless metaphorical use of "family" in naming relationships of all sorts in American culture emerges out of a range of tensions and contradictions I have experienced and observed in my relationship with the man with whom I live. The family construct is often accompanied—even in its Queer versions—by a privileging of image over reality, longevity over functionality, conformity over liberation.[7] As these assumptions and values, which constitute the foundations of even liberal reappropriations of "family," infiltrate all levels and configurations of human relationships, I want to step back and recalculate the gains and losses of this strategy and reconsider whether authenticity, integrity, and freedom can survive the dogged tyranny of the family.

Conflicted feelings about popularized conceptions of relationships and family intrude on my participation in informal, social conversation. What words do I use to designate the man with whom I have lived for the past six years? My confusion here is distinct from liberal gay concerns that words such as "boyfriend," "partner," and "lover" are not imbued with the seriousness, commitment, and concept of permanent bond that people wish to convey. Word choice, to me, seems limited to constructs loaded with problematic meanings. When I refer to him as my "boyfriend," am I indicating that we are in the early throes of dating and romance? By calling him "lover," am I signaling that he is the only person with whom I enjoy intimate sex? Do I have to relinquish the use of the term if we no longer have sex with one another? Is the use of "spouse" tied to images of a folksy, homey life shared by the two of us, with a kettle of soup on the stove and an Irish setter curled up in front of the fireplace? What does "partner" imply about our individuality, independence, and economic organization?

A host of questions are raised in the simple choice of language. In the narrow attempt to name, we also classify, categorize, and draw distinctions. Is this man the center of my universe, or is he one of a dozen individuals whose orbits bring them close to my heart each day? What is it about our spiritual bond that encourages me to distinguish him from friends of two decades? What social forces exist that constitute him as "primary" to me and relegate others to secondary status? How did I come to construct everyday life and a home with him rather than with others?

I know that when I use the term "lover," I participate in a range of social practices—some rebellious and some which reinscribe and fortify the status quo. On one level, I am asserting to a homophobic world that spiritual, sexual, and social bonds may be forged between two bodies gendered as male. At another level, I feel myself proclaiming, "I am loved," "Somebody loves me!" and "I am worthy." I am smugly asserting, "I *have* someone and someone *has* me," "I am part of a unit," and "My loyalties are firmly established."

The highly charged use of "lover" is particularly apparent these days when I first meet a man who arouses desire within me. What meaning will he glean as I drop the term into our initial, casual flirtations? Am I telling him that I am already spoken for, that there are limitations on the possibilities between us? If this man is single, am I suggesting that I am better then he is or that my life is more "together," more worthy? Am I being a tease or simply being candid? Might I be reminding myself that I must rein in initial fantasies of possibilities, or am I deceiving myself about the supposed permanence of my relationship and its imperviousness to external threats?

The tyranny of family intrudes on my everyday conversations in the form of omissions, silences, and distortions of meaning. I speak the word "lover" or "partner" to the world of work, school, and my family of origin, and they hear monogamy, fidelity, and adherence to conventional social formations. Heteronormativity organizes my affections and alliances into a narrow generative mode. I say the word "friend," even "best friend" or "old friend," and they hear "chum" or "buddy." Central discussion of friends is demoted and devalued. I am supposed to see my lover as "primary" and the others as secondary, superficial, and superfluous. In the cinematic version of life, deep experiences of friendship and long histories of connection—social, political, and spiritual—are cast as minor players, members of the chorus, or brief, cameo appearances serving only to foreground the primary relationship. Hence, my most profound interpersonal connections may be misrecognized, miscategorized, and relegated to the junkheap of "old pals."[8]

Literacy, itself, seems unable to be made an ally in expressing the deep and complex affiliations circulating in the social and sexual systems in which we participate. Gay men develop strange bilingual strategic practices, employing one language in the ghetto and another in the mainstream world. Amid heterosexuals, I name the man my "lover," among gay men and lesbians, he is my "husband." Thus we reach an impasse, which is the lot of bicultural people everywhere. We are able to converse in both HetAmeriKa and the Queer nation, but we are at home nowhere.

Why is it easier to be honest about being gay than about participating in gay male culture? Sacred spiritual moments of tribal con-
vocation are euphemized in the mix of public representation.
Spaces that generate ecstatic communal linkages are articulated as
"sex clubs." Moments drawing music and bodies together in rhythmic movement and mass communal celebration are dubbed "dance
parties." A collective social practice exalting joy, desire, and liberation becomes known as a "gay pride parade." How does our choice
of words collapse complexity and trivialize our gatherings? How do
the limitations of diction make pedestrian these core spiritual con-
vergences?

What gets said and what gets silenced when I talk about gay male
cultures with outsiders? I talk with nongay friends and colleagues
about a vacation and describe the beaches, the guest house, even the
food, as if the setting were more important to my enjoyment than
the people. I won't mention the bodies and voices, the hearts and
souls, the smells and the touches of men I enjoyed. I tiptoe around
issues of sexual and spiritual connection beyond my lover and
privatize these dalliances, as if I were shamed by misconduct or
guilty of infidelity. I allow people to cultivate and maintain constricted
visions of gay male culture as hedonistic, facile, and nihilistic by
failing to fully describe my experiences of our communal spaces.

What is spoken and what remains unspoken when we talk about
gay male cultures among ourselves? We employ wholly inadequate
language to represent the complexity of desires and sexual meanings among gay men. When is a "great fuck" more than a discrete
sexual experience? How can words do justice to powerful affirmation and love I share, and a long-term "fuck buddy"? Where do we
voice our esteem for the spaces in which spirit, heart, head, and soul
collide and comingle with sweat and semen?

When male couples go to dinner together, an intricate performance of the institution of the couple is likely to be the unspoken
focus of the evening. We meld the reality of our everyday lives into
the desired family image that we wish to project to a broader world.
Each "husband" and each dyad has mapped out ahead of time the
current landscape of the couple's life together, marking off boundaries, setting aside specific terrain as untouchable, and indicating areas
of contestation. Sometimes this mapping occurs through explicit

conversations; more likely the boundaries of discourse are established through implication, coded gesture, or guiding glances. Although food may fill the table, the meat of the meal is in the construction and affirmation of couple identities through the social practice of dinner conversation.

Hence, a range of remarks, inflections, and gestures come together during the meal to create a paint-by-number portrait of the male couple in the moment. My lover and I may signal devotion to one another by dropping into the conversation a comment on the comfort we find in quiet evenings reading together on the sofa or by a simple and swift touch on the shoulder. The meal unfolds following an agenda that may be read like a list of affirmations of our statuses as husbands: the two couples swap stories of how we met, compare the homes we've created, and talk about pets and children. Middle-class couples may share tips on interior design and home furnishings, career opportunities, pending vacations, and holiday plans. We reaffirm through conversation meaningful situations, symbols, and commodities, which "ark" us as a couple and define the boundaries of what being a couple is allowed to be. Like dancing bears at a circus, performing husbands are meticulously trained to play to a crowd and energetically respond to applause. Thus one couple's amusing and homey story is matched by the other's. In turn, the original couple swiftly generates another anecdote of family life, which is exceeded yet again by an even sweeter story from the second couple.

At times, my lover and I have gone to dinner with other couples and disarmed them with our candor about outside sex, our questioning of the concept of "commitment," and our distinctly antiromantic views of couples. Occasionally, our openness is returned, and we enjoy a powerful and searching conversation among men about the authentic issues we confront in our attempts to come together. More often, however, we are met with stony silence and confused questions. By stepping over the line of acceptable discourse, we are reading from a distinctly unorthodox cultural script, one which might undermine the other couple's usual performance. It is not unusual for us to never again receive an invitation to dine with the couple.

Many of these tensions to perform were experienced when we held a "celebration of love and friendship," after we'd been together for two years. Despite our attempts to distinguish the ceremony from a "gay wedding" (no religious presence, a focus on our friends and family, and our decision not to register as domestic partners at City Hall), many friends insisted on seeing the event as a marriage because our frame of reference is so limited. As we sifted through poems, readings, and songs for the program, we rigorously rejected the bulk of the materials that spoke of such events as "union" and focused on "commitment," "permanence," and "till death do you part." Several years afterward, we attended a ceremony for lesbian friends and caught each other's winks as the couple vowed to be together forever, even in the "afterlife."

Forging a relationship based on honest communication, democratic values, and an openness to life's possibilities has its joys and its challenges. Key to the efforts of my lover and me to "get real" with each other has been a constant scrutinization of the ways in which the culture of romance infiltrates our relationship.

We understand love as a wily social construct loaded with a range of questionable values, and romance as a social practice laden with obligations offered as love letters and power plays masquerading as roses. I am aware that this sounds heartless, but I have participated in enough emotional role-playing in my life, richocheting between being the heel and the jilted lover, to resist the incessant urge for drama in contemporary intimate relations. We have developed our own rituals and symbols to express warmth, acknowledge success, and indicate affection. Yet we engage in active discussion about the meanings we find in these gestures and their relationship to the current dynamics between us. We maintain an amorous relationship marked by humor, shared pleasures, and occasional silliness. Sometimes it works, and sometimes it doesn't, but we don't allow the thick goo of romance to obscure injustices, cover over hurt feelings, or deny boredom.

We have often felt like pioneers as we have embarked on efforts to maintain open and honest communication with each other about outside sexual activities. An early spate of couples' counseling on this topic earned us a shared commitment to full disclosure about each other's sex lives. We call this the "Ask and Tell Policy," and it goes a long way toward maintaining interest and involvement in each other's sexuality, even when mutual erotic play is ebbing. It has led to a diminution of prevarication and deception and a minimizing of sneaking around. As time has gone by, we've developed greater comfort and a broader vocabulary in discussing our outside sex.

Yet a seemingly limitless range of unexpected issues confront all male couples who pioneer various levels of "open" relationships. What does one say on running into one's lover and his "boyfriend" in a restaurant? How does one deal with the feelings of jealousy that arise on seeing a letter arrive from the man your lover tricked with during his recent beach vacation? Is it proper or appropriate to inform a lover that what you really want for your birthday is a rimseat, when both you and he know that rimming has never been his thing?

Finding ways to minimize the level of sexual shame and give ourselves permission to fully probe erotic desire has seemed of primary importance in my relationship. We consider our relationship to be a site we have created in which we can share delights and fears, enjoy common interests and activities, and participate in a deep experience of human growth and change over time. By balancing independence with mutuality, sexual freedom with interpersonal intimacy, and thoughtful communication with occasional frivolity, we aim to find ways to keep the relationship strong and enjoy its continuing evolution.

Gay men's various social formations offer rich opportunities for intimacy and connection free of some of the constrictive features of family life. Although some may wish to shoehorn these formations into definitions of "family," I argue that our attempts to equate childless gay male social formations with even a liberal definition of "family" runs the risk of intermingling constructs with very different values and tainting the creative interpersonal processes used by gay men in constituting relationships. My concern about male couples with children focuses on their tendency to maintain wholly unproblematized understandings of childhood and the traditional use of the nuclear family form to protect, indenture, restrict, and engage in other forms of symbolic violence against children.

Some gay men cite the lack of role models of long-term male couples as oppressive and restricting. I believe the limited visions of emancipatory relationships have forced us gay men, as a class, to draw on our collective imagination in constructing social formations that eschew conformity in favor of liberation. These include not only couples but also trios, groups, and friendship networks. While recognizing the risks and shortcomings of generalizing about gay male social organization, it is clear that several of the most popular options (nonmonogamous couples, sexualized friendship networks, long-distant relationships) challenge key tenets of established family life in America. Among the axioms of family values that we violate are the following popularized beliefs:

Families are forever. Studies show that gay men rarely maintain a single primary relationship throughout their entire lives. More likely, gay men will be participants in several couples throughout their lifetime. Gay men appear more able than others to form a couple when it serves them and leave when needs are no longer being met. This tendency is evident within friendship networks as well. We recognize and anticipate growth and change and jettison longevity in favor of functionality.

The couple is the primary focus for each member's sexuality. Gay male relationships rarely require ongoing sex between partners and frequently, explicitly or implicitly, condone "extramarital" sex. Gay men do not usually require active erotic desire between men to participate in a relationship.

Families are the essential building block of our culture. Despite invitations to black-tie fundraising dinners, which proudly and explicitly link lovers and serve as an annual registry of who's bound to whom, gay men as a class staunchly resist ceding individual autonomy and merging into the melting pot of the couple. Many gay men happily remain single throughout their lives, and many others maintain separate bank accounts, residences, or autonomous lives, even when coupled. Although some may attribute the intransigent individuality and independence to male socialization, regardless of its roots, male couples generally allow one another greater freedom to circulate on their own in public spaces than heterosexual couples, although one study suggests not as much as lesbian couples.[9]

Family members, with the exception of mom and dad, do not have sex with each other. When sex occurs within families, including extended families, power imbalances and role conflicts result in the breakdown of trust and may be experienced as abusive. I am speaking here not of the sexual abuse of children, but of heterosexual husbands and wives sleeping with one another's friends, siblings, and business associates. Television talk shows are populated with every conceivable combination of this sort of infidelity. Yet gay male friendship networks frequently comprise former tricks, current boyfriends, and future lovers. A gay friendship network might include lovers, each of their ex-lovers, a regular fuck buddy of one of the lovers, and a pal who has secretly lusted after the other lover for any number of years. Although abuses of power and privilege certainly can occur within gay male friendship networks, my experience has taught me that more often a friendly, casual playfulness preserves physical and erotic ties between men.

When I look critically at my own life and examine my relationship with my lover, these differences between gay male social formations and families bring ample benefits. We greatly enjoy our time together and work to keep the relationship fresh, intimate, and evolving. However, we are aware that should there come a time when the relationship no longer "works" for either or both of us, and attempts to improve the situation do not work, we may go our separate ways. This may seem cold or callous to state in print because the culture of romance precludes consideration of anything other than permanence. Yet, quite separately, my lover's HIV-positive status serves to force confrontation with questions of longevity, whether we give voice to these possibilities or not. When I think about my life in thirty years, I confront questions about whether or not he will be living.

We also have benefited from vast freedom to explore erotic desires outside our relationship. We do not pretend such activity is unimportant, and we acknowledge the risk outside sex represents. Yet the sexual relationships I've enjoyed with other men have ranged from one-night-only tricks to long-term, loving friendships, which have been sources of tremendous joy and growth for me. By striving to keep sexuality alive between us while supporting each other's outside activity, we've afforded each other a range of possibilities for the creation of meaningful bonds of intimacy and affection within the broader gay tribe.

Currently, we choose to survive without the state's formal participation and intervention in our relationship. The economic costs are tangible. I am not covered by his health plan, nor, because he works for an airline, do I receive free travel benefits, as I would were I to be legally married to him. Yet the cultural and psychic benefits we gain by falling between established categories and social formations make it more than worth the cost. If our resistance to family status does little else than leave us with confusion over word choice and authority over our bodies, we'd choose defiance any day.

NOTES

1. Bruce Bawer, "Family Values Key to Gay Rights." *San Francisco Sentinel*, January 25, 1995, p. 13.

2. Loren King, "Lesbian Journalist Launches Magazine on Gay Family Issues." *Bay Windows*, August 17, 1995, p. 1.

3. Cheryl Deaner, quoted in "1st Family Day Celebration 'In Honor of Families We Have Created.'" *San Francisco Frontiers*, June 8, 1995, p. 55.

4. Lisa Keen, "Wrong Time, Wrong Place: D.C. Gay Marriage Case Ends, and So Does the Relationship." *The Washington Blade*, September 22, 1995, p. 55.

5. Carol Stack struggled with and successfully answered different, though parallel, foundational questions in assessing black kinship networks. See *All Our Kin: Strategies for Survival in a Black Community,* by Carol Stack (Harper & Row, 1974, pp. 30–31).

6. Joseph P. Shapiro, "Heavenly Promises," *U.S. News & World Report*, October 2, 1995, pp. 68–70. See also Larry B. Stammer, "Teaching Patriarchs to Lead," *Los Angeles Times*, June 22, 1994; also Jeff Wagenheim, "Among the Promise Keepers," *New Age Journal*, March/April 1995, p. 78.

7. For a variety of perspectives on contemporary and historical family constructs, see *The Way We Never Were: American Families and the Nostalgia Trap,* by Stephanie Conntz (Basic Books, 1992); *What's Happening to the American Family,* by Sar A. Levitan and Richard S. Belous (Johns Hopkins University Press, 1981); *Domestic Revolutions: A Social Hisotry of American Family Life,* by Steven Mintz and Susan Kellogg (The Free Press, 1988); *Brave New Families,* by Judith Stacey (Basic Books, 1992).

8. *Friends as Family,* by Karen Lindsey (Beacon Press, 1981), offers extensive discussion of the politics, logics, and logistics of families constituted by formations of friends.

9. *American Couples: Money, Work, Sex,* by Philip Blumstein and Pepper Schwartz (William Morrow, 1983), remains to my mind the most interesting snapshot of differences between heterosexual couples (married and unmarried), lesbian couples, and gay male couples.

Chapter 13

Just a Perfect Blendship
Friendship and Sexuality

Elizabeth Stuart

It can be no accident that both Hebrew and Christian writers found the metaphor of marriage an appropriate one for the relationship between God and his chosen people, or the Church. It was a metaphor that conveyed inequality, dominance, and dependence. At the heart of the metaphor is an understanding of marriage very close to slavery.

He plants a cedar and the rain nourishes it. Then it can be used as fuel. Part of it he takes and warms himself; he kindles a fire and bakes bread. Then he makes a god and worships it, makes it a carved image and bows down before it . . . He feeds on ashes; a deluded mind has led him astray, and he cannot save himself or say, "Is not this thing in my right hand a fraud?" (Isaiah 44: 14–15, 20)

One of the positive elements of Catholic Christianity is that it seems to possess a built-in guard against idolatry. The belief in ongoing revelation through the murky windows of a fractured creation prevents the idolization of scripture, which, of course, was formed in much the same way as the wooden idol, which is the subject of Isaiah's exasperation. Some works of human hands were ditched, and some were accepted as sacred. Of course, Catholic Christianity has not been immune from idolatry. Catholics may not have idolized a book, but they have idolized the past, their own constructs of nature, and certain ecclesiastical offices. They have been just as guilty as their Protestant friends of subscribing to what I irreverently call "seagull dropping theology."

We take human institutions and human words and, through some process of collective memory loss, decide that they have actually dropped down from the sky pearly white. This failure to recognize the human construction of theology, despite the efforts of Latin-American, black, Asian, and feminist and womanist theologians to expose the nonneutrality and value-laden nature of "orthodox" Christianity, is still widespread and most clearly demonstrated in Pope John Paul II's recent encyclical on moral teaching, *Veritatis Splendor*.[1] It seems to be a human trait to want to pin God down, to affix her to our human creations like the Victorians affixed butterflies to wooden display cases. But surely the message of the resurrection is that we actually cannot pin God down, that she is, to use R.S. Thomas' words "such a fast God, always before us and leaving as we arrive."[2] This God is not contained, not locked away in books or the past, but blows through our lives, always ahead of us, always summoning us to follow. Neither does she dance in a straight line. She takes us backward, forward, and sideways; she spirals and encircles. When we weave our webs of theology, we are not weaving shrouds to wrap the dead body of God in, nor are we capturing her or sewing her into the patterns we create. In a very real sense, we are weaving the tracks of a God who has already moved on, the trails of the trailblazer. The only reason we speak about God at all is that we see her shadow cast across the faces of people, events, and other things; we smell her perfume on the wind; we see dim echoes of God's image impressed upon the wet clay of our world. All our theology is partial, transitional, and at best but a shadow of the truth. Of course, we have our ancestors in faith to guide, challenge, and cajole us, but they are not God either. Their theology was as partial and transitory as our own.

Exposing and smashing idols has long been a prophetic duty. The place of the prophet is often the place of the marginalized. The space of the marginalized is often a space where imagination can flourish outside the restricting dictates of the mainstream.

Raymond Williams recognized that it is only those whose voices have been drowned out by the dominant culture who will have the motivation to develop a new language, new symbols, and new discourses.[3] The very narrowness of the dominant culture and its discourses leaves plenty of space for such work to be done. What I want to suggest is that in the wake of the International Year of the Family (1994), it might be wise for Christian churches to listen to the voices of those who are widely perceived to be outside of the family unit and threatening to it (including lesbians and gay men) because they may just have some uncomfortable prophetic insight into the whole issue.

The very fact that the family has become such an important political tool should make us suspicious. One of the things we learn about idolatry from the Hebrew scriptures is that it is often bound up with struggles for power and often causes great injustice. It is interesting to observe that an "appropriate" attitude toward marriage and the family has become the ultimate test of orthodoxy in the Church and public life. In Britain, where I live and work, even the leader of the socialist opposition Labor Party feels he has to make the right noises and profess his profound belief in the family. Both Church and government have responded to the current crisis within marriage (in Britain, fewer people are getting married than at any time since World War II) by bribing people into marriage with tax and benefit incentives, the classic capitalist response to everything. We are told by church and State that marriage and the family are the "ideal," created by God as the best means of realizing human potential. Collective amnesia sets in so that we are untroubled by the fact that for most of its history the Church idealized the celibate state, regarding marriage and family life as falling short of the ideal. We are told that we must all sacrifice ourselves to it in one way or another, so that those of us who will not or cannot get married and have children are either supposed to remain celibate (which is the Vatican's teaching) or acknowledge that our relationships "fall short" of this great ideal (which is the Church of England's line).

Like Moses returning to his people at the bottom of Mount Sinai, lesbian and gay people stand on the sidelines of marriage and family life and watch bemused as politicians and clerics lead people to dance around the golden calf and watch with horror as thousands sacrifice themselves to this great beast. Yet, from the outside looking in, marriage and family life are not ideals, particularly for women and children.

The family is the most dangerous place for Western women and children. In Britain, 25 percent of all violent crime is wife assault. Researchers in the United States found that 75 percent of the victims of domestic violence are wives.[4] Overall, the mental health of women deteriorates significantly when they get married, while the mental health of men improves.[5] In Europe, 70 percent of divorces are instigated by women.[6] If any other institution were going so wrong and causing so much pain, one would hope that the Church would be asking some serious questions about it, perhaps even mounting campaigns to rescue people from it. If marriage and family life go wrong, though, it is assumed to be the fault of the people involved and not the fault of the institution. Long ago we convinced ourselves that this was God's creation, and therefore it must be above criticism. Even the briefest dip into the history of marriage reveals that it was constructed to bind women into a particular relationship with men, and that construction still lives on, often masked by the language of equality.

I was horrified when, after a lecture I gave at Manchester University, a group of about eight middle-aged women (most married to clergy) came up to me and said that in the discussion time, they had all revealed to each other that given the chance again they would not get married. Ever since, I have asked every group of mature women I have taught that same question, and many have given the same answer. When I ask, "Why?" the most common response is that they feel marriage has stunted their emotional, intellectual, and spiritual growth. They feel owned. Whenever the issue of cohabitation raises its head in Church circles, the fact that cohabiting couples who subsequently marry are more likely to divorce is often used by those who want the Church to continue to take a judgmental attitude toward cohabitation. What is rarely cited is the evidence that suggests that cohabiting couples demonstrate greater mutuality and equality than married couples.[7] Evidence suggests that once a previously cohabiting couple marry, the man's perception of the woman can change.[8] She becomes his "wife," and he expects her to perform the traditional roles of a wife and mother, as does society at large. This is one reason why cohabiting couples often cannot sustain subsequent marriages.

David Oliphant[9] has drawn attention to the way in which Church and State collude with the extremely lucrative "wedding industry" to obscure the reality of marriage. He has some extremely harsh words to say about the marriage "propaganda" produced by the Church, State, and wedding industry, particularly about marriage's unique suitability as the context for bearing and rearing children:

> I am not sure that marriage and family as we have known and produced it produced the goods in these terms. At best it produced men and women who could continue the traditional social roles, and this on balance gave society a center and a stability. At worst it produced badly damaged people. . . . Any attempt by the Church or any other organization to hang on to old idealism about marriage has got to face and give account of this terrible reality. The depth of woundedness in our society from abuse in families is appalling. At this level traditional marriage has failed to produce reasonably whole and separate adults.

Claiming an institution as God-given and pronouncing forgiveness for those who cannot stay in it excuses the Church from dealing with disturbing facts, and, of course, it is in some people's interests not to deal with reality. Lesbian, gay, and bisexual people, when they live openly outside the institution of marriage, challenge the idol, and that is why we are demonized (along with single mothers).

But what if the outsiders have something to teach the insiders? What if the demons are angels in disguise, and, if so, what is their message?

It would be dishonest of me not to acknowledge that some gay people do define their relationships in terms of marriage and want to be incorporated into the institution of marriage. However, I think it significant that those who have argued this theologically are either gay men or straight men, I have never come across a lesbian theologian arguing for incorporation.[10] Despite the fact that our society only presents us with two models for defining our most intimate, committed relationships—cohabitation or marriage—and the Church only presents us with one, lesbian and gay people have consistently revealed in surveys that they define their primary relationships principally in terms of friendship.[11]

Peter Nardi has explored the meaning of friendship for lesbian and gay people: "Friendship is typically seen as a voluntary, egalitarian relationship, involving personal choice and providing individuals with a variety of psychological, social, and material support."[12] It is the egalitarian nature of friendship that is key here because friendship carries no inherent roles or structures; it is created by the people involved, its boundaries are fluid. It is friendship not marriage that is at the heart of the gospel.

Despite centuries of Christian apologetic to the contrary, it cannot be denied that Jesus' teaching and behavior, as presented to us in the four gospels, is hardly conducive to family life. He is portrayed as demanding that people leave all their social and familial obligations behind them and follow him immediately (Mark 1:16–20). Not even the most sacred familial obligations are considered important enough even to postpone following Jesus (Luke 9:59–62). Jesus is consistently presented as demanding that people deprive themselves of their wealth, status, and home to follow him. In fact, he demands that his disciples learn to "hate" their families (Luke 14:26–27). His attitude toward his own family is consistent with this (Mark 3:31–35). The old bonds of kinship were dissolved and replaced by new ones.

Elisabeth Schussler Fiorenza[13] has drawn attention to the interesting fact that in the Gospels when Jesus speaks about the need to leave behind blood relatives to gain new brothers, sisters, and mothers, he never mentions fathers. *Blood fathers are people to be left behind but not to be replicated in the new order (Mark 19:29–30). No fathers are needed because there is only one father—God. And no fathers are needed because patriarchal structures are antithetical to God's reign.* Virginia Ramey Mollenkott[14] refers to this as God's *kindom,* thereby avoiding the male, monarchical overtones of *kingdom* but still capturing the essence of Jesus' use of *basilea.*

In Mark 12:18–27, Jesus is portrayed in dispute with some Sadducees over resurrection, a possibility the Sadducees rejected. They endeavor to demonstrate the absurdity of the idea by invoking the laws of levirate marriage. In their example, a woman is married seven times to seven different brothers, "In the resurrection whose wife will she be? For the seven had married her," Jesus' reply is clear, "For when they rise from the dead, they neither marry nor are given in marriage, but are like angels in heaven." This is an interesting passage from our point of view because Jesus appears to state clearly that when the glorious reign of God is brought in marriage will no longer exist. This is important because many have interpreted his reference to Genesis 2:24 in his teaching on marriage (Mark 10:2–9) as an expression of a belief that when God's reign came, human beings would be restored to their original married state in paradise.

The mention of angels should not be assumed to be a reference to some kind of sexless state. Jewish understandings of angels were usually very bodily. Indeed, this tradition is continued in the work of John Milton, who has an angel explain to Adam:

> Whatever pure thou in the body enjoy'st
> (And pure thou wert created) we enjoy
> In eminence, and obstacle find none
> Of membrane, joint, or limb. . . . (*Paradise Lost*, VIII, 612–625)

We know that radical reworking of notions of family operated in the early Church. Rosemary Radford Ruether,[15] in surveying the effect of Christianity on the family, has noted the following:

> Christianity disrupted the family, because household and state were so closely linked in ancient society. To follow a religion contrary to that of the family—a religion, moreover, which declared the official religion to be false and demonic—was to strike at the heart of the social order of both the family and the state. It meant that wives could dissolve their allegiance to their households, children to their parents, slaves to their masters. These persons, in turn, no longer reverenced the state whose prosperity was founded on the favor of the ancestral gods. Thus we should not minimize the seriousness of the assault on society posed by early Christianity.

It is undoubtedly true that Christianity had particular appeal to women because of this freedom it gave them *from* the family. Many heroic stories survive from the early centuries of Christianity, attesting to the bravery of women who resisted persecution from their families and the state for their new faith. This bravery often united enslaved with free women and rich with poor—an alliance that further exasperated those who regarded Christianity as socially and politically subversive. In the epistles of the New Testament, however, we find evidence of another tradition, which sought to play down the subversive implications of Christianity for the family to gain state tolerance. Paul typically struggles between what he knows are the radical demands of the Gospel and his own conservative instincts, but he tentatively begins to suggest that marriage and the family can be a locus for living out the way of Christ (Ephesians 5:22–33).

Other writers faced with the problem of households divided by Christianity advocate a kind of dualism. A person is inwardly free but must not cause scandal by actually living this freedom. Physical oppression must be accepted for the sake of Christ (1 Peter 2:18, 21; 3:1). This approach is mirrored in early Christian apologetics. This conflict between attitudes toward family life eventually resolved itself into two separate ways of life—monasticism and what Ruether calls "the Christianization of the patriarchal family and the Roman empire"—leaving the family largely unscathed by the radical Christian vision. "By making the Christian egalitarian counterculture a monastic elite, outside of and unrelated to the family, the Christian Church retrenched from the possibility that this radical vision itself could lay claims upon and transform the power relationships of society and family."[16]

Paul Ballard,[17] in a discussion of Christianity and the family, has noted that "The heart of the matter is that the Gospel has burst through the limitations of accepted human relationships." In terms of the family, it means that the covenant of inclusive friendship desacralizes inherited patterns of family to be replaced by universal bonds of kinship.

The Hebrew Scriptures are also actually subversive of modern attempts to idolize the family in terms of married mother and father plus children. Virginia Ramey Mollenkott has identified forty different forms of family "mentioned or implied" in the Hebrew and Christian Scriptures.[18] These include patriarchal extended families;

polygamous marriage; female-headed extended family; single parents and their children; monogamous marriage; cohabitation without marriage; surrogate motherhood; unrelated adults sharing a home; women married by force; cross-cultural adoptive families; cross-class adoptive families; and even "commuter marriages" (Peter traveling around with Jesus, leaving his wife and mother-in-law at home [Matthew 8:14] and Joanna, wife of Chuza, who did the same thing [Luke 8:3])!

The Hebrew and Christian Scriptures actually speak a great deal more accurately and honestly about family life than most Christian churches do. They do not idealize or sentimentalize but present us with a quilt of images, which we can recognize in our own experience of family life and which cry out in defiance of those who seek to claim it as the source and demander of "traditional family values." Jesus' behavior is the most outrageous of all.

The only model of relating that we can definitely see operating in the life of Jesus, as presented to us by the Gospels, is friendship. One could say that the essence of Jesus' ministry was simply befriending—the forming of mutual, equal, loving, accepting, and transforming relationships. The equality dimension is emphasized by Jesus' refusal to make any claims about himself, despite pressure to do so; his refusal to play the "master" role (John 13:1–11); and his constant concern to encourage others to do what he does—teach, preach, heal, and take responsibility for bringing in the reign of God.

Jeffrey John[19] raises some interesting objections to my thesis that lesbian and gay people, in defining their primary relationships in terms of friendship, may offer the heterosexual world a model for redeeming their relationships from injustice—a view I first articulated in *Daring to Speak Love's Name*.[20] He claims there is no scriptural warrant for defining sexual relationships in terms of friendship, for friendship is a qualitatively different relationship than a sexual commitment: "One may have many friends; one may not, within any moral framework which remotely links Christian teaching, have many sexual partners." My reply to Dr. John is that he may be broadly right that the Bible only sanctions sexual behavior within marriage (if we ignore concubines and slaves), but the biblical picture of marriage is not one most Western women would want to idealize. The only time the scriptures present us with a heterosexual relationship based upon mutuality is in the Song of Songs, where the pair are not married. Indeed, Heather Walton[21] argues that this piece of erotic verse, which has sat so uncomfortably in the canon (so uncomfortably that both Jews and Christians had to convince themselves it was actually an allegory of God's relationship with his people, the Church) cannot be used even to legitimize heterosexual relationships:

> The love is certainly heterosexual, there is no question of this, but not straight in a straightforward sort of way. The lovers are more than lovers, they are, or seek to be, brother and sister. They are, or seek to be, twins. . . . The paradigm in the Song is not a continued supposed complementarity of two binary opposite sexes but of an integration or even disintegration of gendered selves. The lovers frequently eat each other, pass into each other, echo each other and an illustration of this is the fact that scholars have disagreed over which lover is speaking when. . . . The binary opposite presuppositions of heterosexuality are not the rules of this game and when those binary opposites are so confounded heterosexuality becomes a redundant category.

It can be no accident that both Hebrew and Christian writers found the metaphor of marriage an appropriate one for the relationship between God and his chosen people, or the Church. It was a metaphor that conveyed inequality, dominance, and dependence. At the heart of the metaphor, in both the Hebrew and Christian Scriptures, is an understanding of marriage very close to slavery. In Hosea 1–3, the woman whom the jealous but faithful husband passionately pursues is an object to be shamed, humiliated, starved, seduced, and reduced to proper passivity. In Paul (I Corinthians 7:3–5), the language of mutual authority obscures notions of ownership, in which the wife will always be disadvantaged because of the web of power relations in which she must exist and which cannot be conveniently unspun in a marriage bed. The marriage model and metaphor may well be important in the Scriptures, and they have become more important through the Church's development of it, but it is simply unacceptable to those who take the pain and struggle of women seriously. If that is the ideal relationship and the most significant clue as to what God is like, then it is no wonder that many women (straight, lesbian, bisexual) and gay and bisexual men have responded with a polite "No thank you," and have gone on their way.

If we believe that sexual relationships should be based upon mutuality and equality (and there are few Christian theologians who would not now at least pay lip service to this idea), we have to look for models of relationship other than marriage in scripture, and we find several in the covenanted same-sex friendship between David and Jonathan, Jesus and his disciples, and Ruth and Naomi. To say that these relationships are not sexual is to take a very narrow, patriarchal, phallocentric definition of sexual. They are passionate, bodily relationships and therefore sexual, even if genitals never clashed.

Perhaps because we are defined by our sexuality, lesbian and gay people are more acutely aware of the part sexuality plays in all our relationships—that it is our embodied passion that incarnates itself in every friendship, although the level of intimacy and its expression will vary. The false dissection of sexuality and its confinement to one particular authorized relationship has served to perpetuate injustice. The confinement of sexual relationships, simultaneously idealized and abhorred, has meant that they are judged by different standards to other relationships. Violence between people who are "just friends" will be seldom tolerated; violence between those who are having a sexual relationship will usually be ignored.

Jeffrey John[22] is not correct in arguing that it necessarily follows that defining primary relationships in terms of friendship means nonmonogamy. Recognizing a continuum of friendship in all our relationships demands that we take responsibility for our actions, that we learn to negotiate our friendships and the level of physical intimacy in them, and that we respect all of our friendships. It recognizes that sexuality is not some irrational, uncontrollable beast that has to be tamed into one relationship but rather is a rational passion that reaches toward others but remains under the control of our will. We take responsibility for our actions on the basis of friendship to ourselves and others. Mere consent, from the perspective of both Christianity and feminism, is not a firm enough rock upon which to build a sexual ethic because it assumes equality. Friendship involves recognizing differences of power and acting appropriately for the sake of justice. It involves balancing the different demands of friendships.

It would be wrong, of course, to imply that lesbian and gay relationships are models of equality and friendship. We are all socialized in a culture that defines sex in terms of domination and submission, and this inevitably has an effect on all of us. However, in choosing simply to define our relationships in terms of friendship, we offer a prophetic critique of marriage and accidentally touch on something at the heart of the Gospel.

I have already demonstrated that the theme of familial subversion is central to the Gospel. This is but a continuance of a consistent but barely recognized theme of sexual subversion, which runs like a wild underground river through the Hebrew Scriptures.

These Scriptures are littered with stories that demonstrate Yahweh's purposes being advanced by deliberate floutings of sexual convention and law—law which it was believed had come from the deity. The Jewish writer David Biale,[23] commenting on the many incidents that involve incest, notes the following:

> All of these stories no doubt preceded the Levitical incest laws by many centuries; what is therefore noteworthy is that they were included in the biblical text. The authors or editors who produced the text were surely aware of the flagrant contradictions between the laws and the narratives, but they must have seen those contradictions as serving an important cultural function. The creation of the Israelite nation was seen by these later authors as a result of the suspension of conventions, a sign, perhaps, of divine favor for a ragtag, ethically mixed people. Far from a disgrace to be hidden, sexual subversion, like the repeated preference for younger over older sons, hints at the unexpected character of God's covenant with Israel.

The story of Ruth fits into this category. Ruth the Moabite, a member of a nation, which, according to Genesis 19:30–38 was the product of an incestuous relationship between Lot and one of his daughters and which, according to Deuteronomy 23:3–4, should not have been allowed into the "congregation of the Lord," manages to secure the birth of a baby who will be King David's grandfather, by defying expected roles and customs. She transgresses the law by uncovering the "feet" (a euphemism for genitals) of her father-in-law's relation, Boaz, in conspiracy with her Israelite mother-in-law, Naomi.

The book can be read in a number of ways. On the one hand, the whole story revolves around an attempt to catch a husband to ensure that the name of a man will continue to live. The story therefore serves to reinforce patriarchy. On the other hand, the story is about a group of powerless women (and childless widows were among the most powerless people in ancient Israel) whose passionate commitment to each other motivates them to take the future into their own hands. The passionate commitment between Ruth and Naomi is described significantly as *davkah bah* (Ruth "clung to Naomi"), which echoes the words of Genesis 2:24: "Therefore a man leaves his father and his mother and clings (*davak*) to his wife, and they become one flesh." It is this relationship between the Israelite mother-in-law and her Moabite daughter-in-law that secures the male lineage, which will result in the birth of the great king. Even the levirate law, which Ruth was endeavoring to fulfill—the law which decreed that the brother of a man who dies childless should marry his widow to ensure the continuation of his brother's name— are a violation of the incest laws found in the book of Leviticus (18:16; 20:21).

What is particularly interesting about most of the stories that deal with sexual subversion in the Hebrew Scriptures is that the deity is apparently absent. "It is as if God must step backstage in order to make space for human actors, and particularly women, to bend social custom and law . . . God's absence implicitly sanctions these inversions and subversions."[24] God is not completely absent, however. Yahweh is not the outside puppet master but actually the love that exists between the people involved. In the Song of Songs, there may be one tiny explicit reference to the deity, which is easy to miss, particularly in the English translation. It comes in Chapter 8, verse 6. The New Revised Standard Version renders this verse as follows:

> Set me as a seal upon your heart,
> as a seal upon your arm;

for love is strong as death,
passion fierce as the grave.
Its flashes are flashes of fire,
a raging flame.

In speaking of the firelike qualities of love, the Hebrew uses the
term *salhebetya,* which means "a flame of *'yah',* or 'Yahweh
flame.'" It is unclear whether the term is comparing the love with
the fire of the deity or whether their love is regarded as being part of
Yahweh's burning love. "God will be between you and me forever," Jonathan said to David (I Samuel 20:42). Such passages may
suggest to us that in matters of personal relationship we should seek
God, not in law, but in the midst of relationship and that we should
not be surprised to find him in the midst of an unlikely relationship.

I am not arguing that marriage is irredeemable. Indeed, we all
know marriages that are good and happy and based upon friendship,
despite the constraints of being made in a culture that does not
equate friendship with marriage. But it seems to me that the gospel
imperative laid upon the Church is to promote not one particular
human institution but friendship in all our relationships. The celibate, the cohabitants, the heterosexual couple who choose to enter a
public covenant, the lesbian and gay partners who do the same, the
parents and children are thus all involved in the same project,
namely, building the kingdom of God on earth. Friendship is such a
multicolored, multilayered relationship that it is very difficult to
idolize or capture. It is an ethic that demands the best from all of us.

Moral philosophers and theologians such as Alasdair McIntyre
and Stanley Hauerwas[25] have argued that part of the problem with
Christian moral discourse is that it is far too centered on acts and on
whether a particular act is right or wrong, and that it has lost all
sense of moral character. They argue that we need to focus on what
is the right moral character, not on whether individual acts are right
or wrong. What if Aristotle in his *Nicomachean Ethics* was right on
at least this point—that friendship is the source of all other virtues
and that we should be concentrating on turning people into friendly
people who want to realize friendship in all their relationships? If
that were the case, then sexual relationships would no longer be
judged according to the criterion of gender but according to whether

they manifest friendship. Sexual relationships would no longer be seen as somehow qualitatively different from other relationships (a view that has led to the toleration of inequality, exploitation, and violence in sexual relationships), but part of the pattern of all our relationships, part of the same project. Lesbian, gay, bisexual, celibate, and heterosexual would be involved in the same project, too—building up friendship in the world. Like Paul, we may find that we end up obeying most of the old law naturally, but some of it will have lost its relevance and power in the face of experience.

In a world in which marriage and family are still defined and experienced as patriarchal and hierarchical, it seems to me to be singularly inappropriate for the Church to talk about itself as family. It is no accident that those churches that delight in claiming themselves as family can be the most hierarchical and exclusive. Despite St. Paul and Graham Kendrick's famous chorus, many of us do not want to be "adopted into the family" of the Father God. We want to be friends, not slaves.

In June 1995 a working party of the Board for Social Responsibility of the General Synod of the Church of England published a report on the family, called *Something to Celebrate: Valuing Families in Church and Society*. Press coverage of the report gave the impression that it was a radical document calling for the acceptance of heterosexual cohabiting and lesbian and gay couples in church life. It is true that the report (which has no ecclesiastical authority) called for the laying aside of the language of "living in sin" when referring to cohabiting couples, acknowledged that lesbian and gay families existed, and argued that both groups should be accorded a warm welcome in church communities. The report even warned against the idolatry of the family and stressed the importance of friendship.[26] However, this pseudoradical language only serves to obscure the same old liberal Anglican approach. Lesbian and gay people, along with cohabiting couples, are people to be welcomed into already existing structures. Their experience is actually not taken seriously at all, as an open paragraph makes clear: "The vision of the Report is to affirm marriage as the basic framework." Indeed on the subject of cohabitation, the report encourages the Church to see the popularity of this form of bonding "as an opportunity and a challenge to the Church to articulate its doctrine of marriage in ways so compelling . . .

that the institution of marriage regains its centrality." Scripture and tradition are read as being almost entirely family and marriage friendly, and Jungian notions of the masculine and feminine are used uncritically in support of heterosexual marriage. The report concludes with a list of recommendations to the Church and the nation. Lesbian and gay people only figure into one of the recommendations, and even then it isn't really a recommendation: "We welcome continuing discussion on issues related to gay and lesbian people and urge that this take place in a spirit of openness and generosity." Lesbian and gay employment, housing, adoption, and health concerns are nowhere even acknowledged. The nation is not encouraged to examine its homophobic structures and laws. For lesbian and gay people, there is nothing to celebrate in this report.

Lesbian, gay, and bisexual people expose the social construction of our human relationships. These were built by our own hands; they did not drop from the metaphorical sky. They are not as natural as the sheep in the field and the birds in the trees. We may well detect the perfume of God within them; we may detect the shadow of God across the faces of those involved, to use traditional language. God may bless, but don't blame her for the creation. Christians believe in being born again, in resurrection, that it is possible to refashion and reconstruct human relationships. This is indeed what Christianity is all about. The tragedy is that golden calves are so much easier to manage than a God who disturbs, dances, and resurrects.

A nineteenth-century American feminist once commented that there would be no marriage in heaven because there would be no men there! Perhaps there will be no marriage in heaven because there will be no straight people there. I do not mean that those who have lived a heterosexual lifestyle will be turned away at the pearly gates, but if the hunch of lesbian and gay theologians is correct, and the kingdom of God is essentially Queer, i.e., subversive of all attempts to divide and order people into unequal power relations and circumscribe their relationships, then there will be no barriers at all to relating justly, intimately, and bodily with each other. Until, like the nineteenth-century novelist and cleric, Charles Kingsley, we are comfortable with the idea of sex in heaven (however we understand that concept), we will reveal ourselves to be still gripped by the icy hand of body- and sex-hating dualism that lies at the heart of homophobia.

Lesbian, gay, transgendered, and bisexual people Queer the pitch of the theological tradition that idolizes marriage and family life. We incarnate and sacramentalize the kingdom of God, which Cole Porter summed up so lyrically:

It's friendship, friendship,
Just a perfect blendship.

NOTES

1. *Veritatis Splendor* by Pope John Paul II (Catholic Truth Society, 1993).

2. *Pilgrimages*, by R.S. Thomas (London: Macmillan, 1978).

3. *Problems in Materialism and Culture: Selected Essays*, by R. Williams (Verso and New Left Books, 1980).

4. *Distorted Images: Christian Attitudes to Women, Men, and Sex*, by A. Borrowdale (London: SPCK, 1991).

5. *The End of Marriage: Why Monogamy Isn't Working*, by J. Hafner (Century, 1993).

6. *Reconstructing Family Values*, by A. Borrowdale (SPCK, 1994).

7. *Cohabitation*, by K. Kiernan and V. Estaugh (Family Policy Studies Centre, 1993).

8. *Marriage Inside Out: Understanding Problems of Intimacy*, by C. Clulow and J. Mattison (New York: Penguin, 1989).

9. "Marriage: A Union of Equals?" by D. Oliphant, 1991 Mary Body Memorial Lecture, *St. Mark's Review*, Autumn.

10. *Toward a Theology of Lesbian and Gay Marriage*, by R. Williams (Anglican, 1990); *Liberating Sex: A Christian Sexual Theology*, by A. Thatcher (London: SPCK, 1993).

11. "Permanent Partner Priorities: Gay and Straight," by M.R. Longer, in *Gay Relationships*, edited by J.P. DeCecco (Binghamton, New York: Harrington Park Press, 1988); *Identities in the Lesbian World: The Social Construction of Self*, by B. Ponse (Greenwood Press, 1978); *The Lesbian Couple*, by D.M. Tanner (D.C. Heath, 1978).

12. "That's What Friends are for: Friends as Family in the Gay and Lesbian Community," by P. Nardi, in *Modern Homosexualities: Fragments of Lesbian and Gay Experience*, edited by K. Plummer (London: Routledge, 1992).

13. *Discipleship of Equals: A Critical Feminist Ekklesia-logy of Liberation*, by Elisabeth Schussler Fiorenza (London: SCM, 1993).

14. *Sensuous Spirituality: Out from Fundamentalism*, by V. R. Mollenkott (Crossroad, 1993).

15. "An Unrealised Revolution: Searching Scripture for a Model of Family," by R. Radford Ruether, in *Christianity and Crisis: A Christian Journal of Opinion*, vol 43, p. 400.

16. Ibid., p. 400.

17. "The Social Context of the Family Today: A Christian Reflection" by P. Ballard, in *Contact*, No. 114, p. 11.

18. *Sensuous Spirituality: Out from Fundamentalism*, by V.R. Mollenkott (New York: Crossroad, 1993).

19. *Permanent, Faithful, Stable: Christian Same-Sex Partnerships*, by J. John (London: Affirming Catholicism, 1993).

20. *Daring to Speak Love's Name: A Gay and Lesbian Prayer Book*, by E. Stuart (London: Mowbray, 1995).

21. "Theology of Desire," by Heather Walton, in *Theology and Sexuality*, no. 1, 1994, pp. 31–41.

22. *Permanent, Faithful, Stable: Christian Same-Sex Partnerships*, by J. John · (London: Affirming Catholicism, 1993).

23. *Eros and the Jews: From Biblical Israel to Contemporary America*, by D. Biale (New York: Basic Books, 1992), p. 17.

24. Ibid., p. 17.

25. *Character and Christian Life: A Study in Theological Ethics*, by S. Hauerwas (Trinity University Press, 1975).

26. *Something to Celebrate: Valuing Families in Church and Society*, by the Working Party of the Board for Social Responsibility (Church House Publishing, 1995). All other citations in this paragraph are from this source.

Chapter 14

Making Love for the Whole World to Feel
Four Erotic Rituals for Gay Men

Joseph Kramer

Each sacred brother has equal access to the cocreated erotic force field that results each day from 16 men consciously generating the highest fire possible in a human being. Sacred brothers often report that they are vibrated by this energy into transpersonal and mystical states. Most agree that this energy brings them clarity and generosity about the gifts they carry for others. Some sacred brothers impregnate the collective erotic fire with their individual intentions, often with extraordinary results. In some rituals, the whole community agrees to hold the same intention in their hearts. Often when a sacred brother is sick, he will request that he be able to sit or recline in the middle of the omega realm. The erotic vibrations of the community can then swirl around him and through him, shifting and transforming the vibratory patterns of disease to those of well-being. Although the ritual seldom involves ejaculation, when a sacred brother is sick, it is common practice for others to anoint him with their semen. Many of the sacred brothers have expressed their desire to die in the ritual space, bathed, nourished, and blessed by the communal heart fire.

As we approach the year 2000, tens of millions of human beings in the United States have lost their zest for life. As one Queer San Francisco taxi driver put it, "Follow my bliss? I can't even find neutral. The old story of how I live my life—how I eat and sleep and fuck and dream—no longer works." Gay men and lesbians in great numbers are languishing because they have not found the appropriate environments in which to be fully human and share their gifts with others. What do we need to grow into wholeness and to live up to our full spiritual potential? My deepest visions focus on a new monasticism. We need to find or create less toxic and more nourishing environments.

When I was seventeen years old, I left my parents and my life as a marathon masturbater to join the Society of Jesus, a Roman Catholic community, also known as the Jesuits. I embraced totally the Jesuit ideal: "To be man for others." For the next ten years, I never doubted that I was meant to live in a community of men dedicated to service. The question I did ponder in my personal discernment and in my interactions with my spiritual counselors was "Do I have the gift of celibacy?" The Roman Catholic Church and the Jesuits taught that a man "called" to be a Jesuit has to live his whole life without engaging in any sexual activity, including masturbation. Furthermore, a Jesuit was prohibited from consciously thinking erotic thoughts.* If a man could walk this sexless, religious path without serious negative consequences, he was said to possess the gift of celibacy.

Although I rejoiced that the Society of Jesus was a Christian, homosexual environment with most of my fellow seminarians and my Jesuit advisors and teachers being men who loved men, I painstakingly came to realize that the Jesuits were not the best community of men for me. I didn't have the required gift of celibacy. At twenty-eight years old, I finally acknowledged that my special way of loving and serving others involved the gift of my sexuality.

During my seminary years, I witnessed an astonishing tragedy. The majority of Jesuits I encountered were struggling to pursue their spiritual path with integrity but without the so-called gift of celibacy. Their fear and suppression of eros generated enormous personal and societal dysfunction. Candor and intimacy, trust and mutual support became impossible. My experience in the Jesuits taught me that the denial of the gift of sexuality is a denial of God's grace. My rejection of my special way of loving was the "sin against the Holy Spirit," the only sin that cannot be forgiven. I had no choice but to leave the Jesuits. My life's commitment then became a journey to find or to cocreate a community of men whose justice-doing and lovemaking were gifts for the world.

My search led me through the gay sexual undergrounds of New York and San Francisco; into the woods with the Radical Faeries;

---

*Actually, the Roman Catholic church teaches that all Catholics must be celibate, except married couples who are preparing to procreate.

and across the Pacific to Centerpoint, the "free sex" community of New Zealand. I researched the history of orgies, the Knights Templar, the O.T.O. Eleventh Degree, the Cathars, shamanism, peyote sex rituals, Taoist and Tantric sex, and the Oneida Community. In my search I came across many gay communities, but none had both the degree of commitment I sought or the erotic rituals that celebrated what Whitman called the "dear love of comrades."

After twenty years of research into the ways that men who love men could live, I now believe that 20 percent of gay and bisexual men can only realize their human potential in some dynamic form of communal living. In other words, 20 percent of men who love men are extremely frustrated in the present moment with their perceived options. I believe another 50 percent of gay and bisexual men would profit greatly from living a year or more in an erotic-spiritual community. In the monasteries I envision, the monks enact rituals that cocreate an erotic vibratory force field that wakes up the fullness of being human and unleashes our gifts for the community and the world.

In this essay I share four body-based sex rituals I have developed for groups of gay and bisexual men.* In describing three of the rituals, I have made up fictional situations that I hope are useful to you in your visualizing and understanding. I wish to thank the ten thousand men who have ecstatically participated with me in the development of these four rituals. I sincerely hope that the descriptions of these ceremonies motivate you to try them or to create your own.

RITUAL 1
Group Oil Massage: A True Story

On my birthday in 1983, a dozen of my friends and lovers, my chosen family, shared a meal with me. My after-dinner speech went something like this: "Over the years, you have all touched me deeply. You have helped me grow into who I am. Tonight I would like to experience your collective touch. And I would like you to feel who I have become." My massage table always graced my

---

*Although the initial goal of my research was to create ways that helped queer men celebrate the wildness, the mystery, and the nurturance of our sexuality, these rituals have been used by groups of men and women and by groups of women alone.

living room. I gave out several bottles of warm oil, shed my clothes and climbed onto the table. What I thought would last ten minutes went on for well over an hour. I could feel this touch was different from any massage I had ever received. This communal touch of my family celebrated my coming into a body. I was renewed. I have not found a better birthday ritual.

A few months later, I began offering this experience to groups of gay and bisexual men, first in my home and then every Sunday night at my massage school. Fifteen to forty men showed up every week for eight years; over 7,000 men have participated in this ritual. The three-hour experience started with each man greeting every other man with several deep breaths while looking in his eyes. There were verbal introductions, much laughter, some stretching, and tender caresses. Everyone then took off his clothes, and men gathered four to each massage table, where each man received 30 minutes of massage from his comrades. The man on the table directed his massage, instructing his masseurs where and how he wanted to be touched. If the man on the table requested that his genitals be massaged, the masseurs were encouraged to touch with the intention of waking up, pleasuring, and healing, not with the goal of making him ejaculate. During the eight years I experimented with group oil massage, more men requested special attention to their necks and shoulders than asked for genital touch.

At the end of the night, after all four men had been massaged, we would stand in a circle, naked, relaxed, tired, and grateful for this embodied way to be with each other. This was not a celebration of an existing community, but over months and years, the ritual helped foster community bonds among hundreds of men in Oakland and Berkeley.

In the fall of 1995, I was invited to guide a group of gay and lesbian Catholic workers in a group oil massage evening. These Queer Christian anarchists and activists had gathered for a week of spiritual retreat, traveling to Oakland from their local communities all over North America. These "friends of Dorothy," known for justice-doing and serving the poor, were not totally comfortable with the idea of a naked group massage. I asked them, "Will there ever be a safer, more loving group to lay hands on you than these, your fellow gay Catholic workers?" Everyone chose to participate.

Two men, honoring their comfort level, decided not to remove all of their clothes. In the days following the ritual, most of the group acknowledged that the physical intimacy of group oil massage had opened them to new dimensions of community that they had not previously experienced.

RITUAL 2
Soloving: Night Moves to Weave Body, Mind, and Spirit—A Useful Fiction

As another day comes to an end, the monk prepares for his nightly ritual.* He takes deep, comfortable breaths as he warms the coconut oil, moves the massage table aside, and spreads his grandmother's patchwork quilt on the floor in front of the wall mirror. He selects a tape of slow, rhythmic chants. He lights candles as he begins to breathe with the music, effort on the inhale, relaxing on the exhale.

This is the night of the great slowdown. In recent weeks, the ritual has seemed to lose its power. Overwhelmed by grief and plagued by a growing number of distractions, the monk has had trouble focusing his awareness. On some nights he had shortened the ritual, jerked off, and gone to bed. On other nights he couldn't even masturbate. "Slow down the speed of your self-touch," his spiritual advisor had suggested, "and remind yourself again and again of your intentions."

After circling the room, burning some sage he had gathered in New Mexico, the monk stands in the flickering candlelight, looking at himself in the mirror. He feels his chest swell with each inhale and his muscles relaxing on the exhale. He begins to speak his intentions.

> I breathe for myself. I breathe to nourish every level of my being. I breathe to wake up. And I breathe for loved ones who no longer breathe, especially Darrell, Michael, David Christopher, and Grandma.

---

*"Soloving" is a word I created because I was disenchanted with the term "masturbation." I combined the words "solo" and "loving."

As he takes off his clothes, he watches himself in the mirror. He laughs, amazed at how different he feels without clothes. He rubs his hands together, then reaches his palms toward his double in the mirror.

> I offer my hands for the waking of the whole universe. I offer my hands for the healing of those I serve. I offer my hands for the pleasuring of this body.

His strong masseur's hands, so skilled at touching others' bodies, now slowly begin to caress his own naked flesh. His fingertips brush across nerve endings from feet to head and down again. In recent weeks, he has been practicing giving and receiving touch at the same time.

The monk now begins several minutes of shaking every part of his body. The movement, gentle at first, becomes progressively more chaotic.

> I let go; I surrender.
> I let go of how I think this meditation should be.

And then the naked man begins to stretch aliveness into his neck and shoulders. With one breath for each turn, he rolls his neck a dozen times in one direction, then a dozen deep breaths in the other direction. He begins to allow sounds to escape on the exhale. He rolls his shoulders forward until the breath and the movement are one. Up the back on the inhale, down the front on the exhale. He then reverses direction. As he continues to stretch other muscle groups, his awareness focuses on the tinglings and vibrations in his hands, wrists, lips, and thighs. His groans of release transform into moans of aliveness. The thoughts of the day have become silent.

> Happy and aligned with the One are those who find their home in the breathing.[1]

The monk, his breath still dancing with the music, looks at his naked double in the mirror. With his palms together at his heart, he bows, honoring the man he sees reflected. His gaze moves from his heart area down to his genitals and back again. He lets his eyes shift to soft focus as he pours oil into his hands. It is time to anoint—slowly, ever so slowly—the places from which his love flows.

> As I consciously and lovingly touch my body, so I touch with awareness and love the whole universe.

Warm palms rub warm oil into heart, into genitals. Then the monk slows his breathing, stops massaging, one hand resting on his heart, the other cupping his genitals. He again prays, touching the places of love.

> As I receive pleasure, so the whole universe receives pleasure through me.

He now begins his nightly dance, massaging his genitals, his heart and the pathway between. His breath quickens.

> When I'm hard, I remember my heart.
> When I'm hard, I remember my belly.
> When I'm hard, I remember to breathe.
> When I'm hard, I remember my feet,
> When I'm hard, I remember my asshole.

The monk chants his litany, stroking his magic wand with one hand, generating enormous amounts of erotic energy. The other hand massages this sacred nourishment to every part of his body. Remembering his spiritual director's wisdom, he keeps his strokes slow, avoiding the male impulse to beat faster, to rush to climax.

> When I'm hard, I remember my mom and dad.
> When I'm hard, I remember my ancestors.
> When I'm hard, I remember lovers and friends.
> When I'm hard, I remember those who come to me for touch.
> When I'm hard, I remember to ask for help.
> When I'm hard, I remember to be thankful.
> When I'm hard, I remember to be silent.

Laughing at the wonder of it all, the monk massages himself, breathing and dancing. After five minutes or thirty minutes, when his body tells him to slow down his dance, he takes a deep breath and holds it in, clenching all the muscles of his bliss-filled body. He stretches his arms to the sky, ten seconds of clenching, twenty seconds, thirty seconds. His lungs explode into breathing. Some nights, at this point in the ritual, he collapses to the floor, losing normal consciousness. But tonight he remains standing, a little wobbly, looking in the mirror. What he sees—swirling images, bright colors, impenetrable shadows—hardly looks like a man. And then the image in the mirror fades. He sees nothing.

> When I'm hard, I expect visions.
> When I'm hard, I remember my death.
> When I'm hard, I remember love.
> When I'm hard, I am embodied.

The monk finishes his soloving ritual with a few minutes of sitting quietly. He then wipes the oil from his body with no words or thoughts, just quiet breaths. He blows out the candles, and he is ready for sleep.

RITUAL 3
Heart Fire: A Fiction

Jeffrey walks the two blocks from his apartment to the Kiva for the morning ritual. It has been almost a year since he joined the village, a community of sixteen men committed to cocreating, containing, and circulating an "erotic vibratory force field for healing, nourishment, and consciousness." Some community members live together; others, like Jeffrey, live by themselves. All live within a few blocks of the big house and the Kiva. Presence at the daily Heart Fire Ritual is central to being a part of the village. The community members call each other "sacred brother."

Very quickly Jeffrey discovered that being present at the ritual took preparation. Within a month of his acceptance into the village, his whole day revolved around the ritual. He intensified his stretching and exercising, more aware each day of new levels of feeling. He stopped eating and drinking what wasn't nourishing. He seldom watched television and stopped reading newspapers completely. He even started to enjoy his work at the testing center at the university.

For the first time in his life, he felt he was developing relationships—with himself, with his sacred brothers, and with the whole universe. And now, after almost a year of rituals, he feels and understands his life in terms of energy. Jeffrey, the erotic physicist, has learned how to generate energy, contain it, circulate it, focus it, and transmit it. Every day he celebrates the power and the mystery of eros, the evolutionary thrust. Most amazing to Jeffrey, he has discovered a sense of wonder and awe that often allows him to laugh and cry at the same time. Such are the effects of the ritual.

Not a traditional Native American Kiva, the Village Kiva is a Buckminster Fuller-type geodesic structure, containing one huge room about twenty-five feet in diameter, half in the earth, half above ground. The very top of the dome is glass; the wooden polygon sides provide privacy. An elevated platform, three feet high and three feet wide, circles the edge of the room. Candles are everywhere.

Jeffrey usually gets to the Kiva a bit early. Leaving his clothes in the antechamber, he picks up two towels and some massage oil. He spreads one towel on the rug at his favorite place on the platform and prepares to enter void, one of the three realms participants can move among during the ritual. Some sacred brothers jokingly call this realm "voyeur" because it is about doing nothing, just being with the energy of the ritual and witnessing what is happening. Those in void sit quietly on the platform. The heart fire ritual begins and ends with all participants in void.

The second realm of the ritual dance concerns the great human venture of waking up. This is the realm of shaking and stretching, laughing and screaming, self-massage and aerobic activity, breathing, and masturbating. Remaining within his own segment of the platform, each sacred brother generates and circulates within his body the holy fire, the erotic life force, the *ching chi*.* Having spent most of the rituals of the last year in dance, Jeffrey is totally comfortable stretching, stroking himself, and screaming both in pleasure and pain. He often tells others that one of the great delights of the ritual is watching the circle of men he has grown to love wake

---

Ching chi is a Taoist sexual term for erotic life force energy that we feel as sexual pleasure. More explanation of the term and Taoist sexuality is available in the description of the Taoist Erotic Massage Ritual.

up while he, too, wakes up alongside them. Jeffrey has learned to model and imitate the best and most effective of his sacred brothers' movements and rhythms. In dance, everyone is teacher and guide to everyone else.

When the physical, energetic body is sufficiently awakened, a sacred brother can move down into the center of the Kiva. Omega is the realm of joyous movement, ecstasy, celebration, aliveness, communion, glowing eroticism, emptiness, and fullness, synergy, creativity, magi, and mysticism. During the ritual, the center of the Kiva seems to be a place beyond choosing. Most sacred brothers are surprised to find themselves in omega.

The heart fire ritual, usually an hour long, has no leader, only a timekeeper who also plays the music. Sacred brothers can choose at any time to move from one realm to another that seems more appropriate. Often, one or more sacred brothers will sit for the whole ritual in void. It is not uncommon for some sacred brothers to change realms ten or twenty times during a ritual. His second time in omega, Jeffrey was receiving wild erotic touch from a group of sacred brothers when he got distracted by a desire. "I want this in my bed every night," he thought. This thought pulled him out of the present away from one of the hottest experiences of his entire life. He was now *thinking* instead of *experiencing*. He knew he needed to shift to dance to get out of his mind. He gently extricated himself from the scene and returned to his place on the platform.

Each sacred brother has equal access to the cocreated erotic force field that results each day from sixteen men consciously generating the highest fire possible in a human being. Sacred brothers often report that they are vibrated by this energy into transpersonal and mystical states. Most agree that this energy brings them clarity and generosity about the gifts they carry for others. Some sacred brothers impregnate the collective erotic fire with their individual intentions, often with extraordinary results. In some rituals, the whole community agrees to hold the same intention in their hearts. Often when a sacred brother is sick, he will request that he be able to sit or recline in the middle of the omega realm. The erotic vibrations of the community can then swirl around him and through him, shifting and transforming the vibratory patterns of disease to those of well-being. Although the ritual seldom involves ejaculation, when a sacred brother is sick, it is common practice for others to anoint him with their semen. Many of the sacred brothers have expressed their desire to die in the ritual space, bathed, nourished, and blessed by the communal heart fire.

Remarkable relationships develop within the context of the ritual. Two sacred brothers, in particular, function unwittingly as temple dancers for Jeffrey. Authentic temple dancers are men and women who consciously witness to what is humanly possible through their graceful movement and high levels of erotic vibration. These two sacred brothers make Jeffrey rock hard when he focuses on them in dance. When either or both of them are in omega, Jeffrey falls into a love trance where he opens his heart to the whole universe. Jealousy is not a major problem in the village, probably because each member generously makes himself and his gifts available to the rest each day in the ritual.

Each week, the village has a two-hour gathering to talk about the ritual. The following are some of the sacred brothers' reflections:

> We should invite visitors more often. They stimulate us out of our normal patterns and help celebrate diversity. Response: But some are unconscious vampires, totally unaware of the subtlety of what we are doing.

> After charging my body with breath and sex, I often travel to other domains. My body is the gateway, but when I let go into another consciousness, I realize I am not present in the ritual so I come back, but I am frustrated. If my body is the gateway, why not honor it as that. Why commit to staying present with the body for the whole hour?

> I believe that it is possible for us to have as much influence on the world with the heart fire ritual as did Gandhi or Martin Luther King, Jr.

> Whenever I am touching any of you in omega, I feel like I am touching myself.

> My heart keeps getting bigger and bigger. I want to thank each of you. I used to hold back part of my heart waiting for the relationship that would last forever. Now I know that when I

truly love someone, that love is outside of time—forever. This is what I have always wanted but couldn't visualize clearly.

I would like to try a twenty-four-hour version of the ritual.

Why don't we each write a special intention on cards that we place face down in the center of the floor before the ritual. When we are ecstatically moving in omega, we can each pick up a card and focus on that intention.

My boyfriend and I have been doing the ritual together, just the two of us. I love to sit in void and watch him get charged.

Last week I sat in void for six days. I know some of you are concerned. I would like to read a few words from Walt Whitman's "Song of Myself": "I exist as I am, that is enough. If no other in the world is aware, I sit content. And if each and all be aware, I sit content."

RITUAL 4
Taoist Erotic Massage: Another Fiction

"Arousing the Genitals of Christ" was the theme for a men's retreat at our Metropolitan Community Church in 1991. Because many in the congregation felt that the topic was inappropriate, even sacrilegious, the gathering was only half full. Those men who chose to attend invited God into realms where many in the church felt he had no business being, and thus they experienced a "holy instant," an integration of their sexuality and their spirituality. Such is the power of the genitals of Christ.

The following is the invitation to the three-day retreat, including a quote from St. Paul:

If your whole body was just one eye, how would you hear anything? If it was just one ear, how would you smell anything? Instead of that, God put all the separate parts into the body on purpose. If all the parts were the same, how could it be a body? As it is, the parts are many but the body is one. The eye cannot say to the hand, "I do not need you." nor can the head say to the feet, "I do not need you." If one part is hurt, all parts are hurt with it. If one part is given special honor, all parts enjoy it. Now you together are Christ's body; but each of you is a different part of it. (1Cor 12:17–21, 26–27, Jerusalem Bible). Some men who love men are the eyes of the body of Christ. Our visions educate and offer guidance to the community. Some of us are the hands of Christ. Our touch is healing and sought after. But what about those of us who are called to be the genitals of Christ?[2] Let us both individually and collectively reclaim our erotic gifts and make them available to a sexually wounded and erotically malnourished society.

The Mystical Body Monastery was birthed during that retreat. Six men committed to live together to explore the vocation of generating erotic energy within and for the body of Christ. Today, in an apartment building near the MCC church, twelve of us live in relationship, "making love for the whole body to feel." No, we don't have sex all day long. In fact, two of us work at the church, and three of us work with AIDS agencies. Most men kept the same jobs they had before they joined the Mystical Body. There is one couple in the monastery. One man is on disability; one is retired. Half of us are HIV positive. We see our relationships with one another as central to our spiritual path.

I would like to describe to you the favorite ritual of our monastery, Taoist erotic massage. At least once a week, each monk both gives and receives this sacred touch.

The Taoist approach to sex has been foundational for the erotic rituals of our monastery. Taoism is a Chinese cosmology that perceives the universe as energy constantly changing. According to Taoist sexual teaching, when a man's "jade stalk" is stimulated, an astonishing energy called *ching chi* is unleashed in the body. This erotic life force is felt as pleasure, as an intense aliveness, and as vibrancy. When this sacred energy circulates through the heart, it becomes compassion.

By giving and receiving Taoist erotic massage, we are committed to nourishing with *ching chi* all realms of being, every level of self. The monk receiving the massage breathes in a variety of rhythmic patterns, which helps him stay in the present moment. The breathing also helps keep the musculature of his body relaxed, even during high erotic states, and circulates the ching chi. Often, the monk, consciously breathing throughout his massage, experiences a breath orgasm in his body similar to an erotic orgasm. When a "yin" breath orgasm and a "yang" erotic orgasm happen simultaneously in the body, the ego begins to dissolve, and expanded levels of consciousness are possible. In the monastery, we call this state, "the Great Alleluia."[3]

The Taoist distinction between ejaculation and orgasm has been helpful to us in our erotic ceremonies. Ejaculation is a physical act, propelling semen out of the body; this most often discharges energy. Orgasm is an intense, pleasurable, energetic feeling-state in the body. The Great Alleluia occurs when the sexual feelings and the breath feelings intensify to such a degree that we become one with the vibration. Our experience is that the energy is easily transmitted by each monk's intentions and certainly by the prayers of the whole community. In this mystical, orgasmic state, the monk often cannot tell if he has an erection or not, nor can he tell if he has ejaculated or not. We offer the energy we generate during the Great Alleluia for the waking and nourishing of the whole body of Christ.

Usually a monk fasts or only drinks fresh juices the day before he receives a Taoist erotic massage. He sleeps that night, not in his own room, but on a massage table in a warm meditation chamber. Naked under a blanket, he sleeps on his side or his stomach, making his back available to be touched first. Before he sleeps, he renews his commitment as the genitals of Christ to the waking and nourishing of the whole body. The monk then prays for visions and dreams for himself and for all his fellow monks.

His masseur, chosen by lot, rises toward the end of night. After breathing and stretching his body awake, the masseur sits in silent meditation for twenty minutes. Then one hour before sunrise, he quietly enters the meditation room. Reaching his warm hands under the blanket, he begins to caress and vibrate the back muscles of the sleeping monk. For the next half hour, the masseur works along the bladder meridian, a pathway of energy stretching from the head to the little toe. He begins with light fingertip brushes, slowly progressing to rather intense deep-tissue massage of the muscles of the back. As the monk wakes up, he begins to breathe consciously. Many in the monastery have cultivated the skill of remaining in a sleep state while aware of being touched. Two of the monks have even learned to speak aloud their dreams and visions to their masseurs before waking up.

For the second half hour, the masseur invites the man receiving to turn over onto his back. The breathing becomes deeper and sometimes faster. The masseur begins to stimulate the places of love, the heart and the genitals. Like all the monks at the Mystical Body, he knows over a hundred different ways to pleasure the jade stalk.[4] After only fifteen minutes of erotic touch and ecstatic breathing, most monks let go into the Great Alleluia.

At sunrise, after half an hour of muscle massage and another half hour of erotic touch, the masseur stops and removes his hands from the electric body. He guides his fellow monk in "the big draw," a clenching of muscles and a holding of breath that thrusts the orgasmic energy up through the central core of the body, through the heart and out the top of the head. Often the big draw deepens and lengthens the Great Alleluia. Then both giver and receiver remain in the chamber for another half hour. The ritual officially ends when the masseur towels the oil from the man on the table. He records in a notebook any observations or images voiced by the man who received his touch, and he then adds his own awarenesses. I am happy to report that it is becoming more common for the Great Alleluia to extend beyond the ritual into the daily lives of the monks of the Mystical Body.

I align myself with the school of cultural anthropologists who believe that the evolutionary leap from primate to human happened because of the anatomical ability of primates to look in each other's eyes during sexual orgasm. This face-to-face ecstasy pushed us to new levels of consciousness. We are in dire need of another evolutionary leap, which I believe has to do with communally created erotic vibratory force fields. As individuals, we don't have the ability to create the fire necessary for the growth in consciousness. I believe that one of the social roles of gay men is to be consciousness scouts, exploring what is erotically possible.

NOTES

1. This is Neil Douglas-Klotz's translation of Matthew 5:3 from his book *Prayers of the Cosmos: Meditations of the Aramaic Words of Jesus*, Harper & Row, Publishers, San Francisco, 1990, p. 47.

2. Heterosexuals called to be the genitals of Christ offer a needy world nourishing love, often in the form of children. For a different perspective on the genitals of Christ, see my video lecture. *Male Sacred Prostitutes: An Ancient Spiritual Path for Today* (50 minutes), EroSpirit Research Institute, P.O. Box 3893, Oakland, CA 94609.

3. "The Great Alleluia" is a term that was coined by Dan Bredemann, an ex-Jesuit, erotic evolutionary, writer, and healer.

4. For instruction in over thirty ways to massage the jade stalk, see my video *Fire on the Mountain: An Intimate Guide to Male Genital Massage* (45 minutes), EroSpirit Research Institute, PO Box 3893, Oakland, CA 94609.

Chapter 15

"Where Two or More Are Gathered"
Using Gay Communities as a Model for Christian Sexual Ethics

Kathy Rudy

This emphasis on monogamy, I suggest, urges gays to mimic heterosexual relational structures. We are told that on the deepest level our allegiance and commitment belong not to our larger community but to our partner or nuclear family. We are encouraged to participate in the American dream by buying a house and living "together," i.e., to separate ourselves from larger kinship systems. While living in this nuclear unit, we are encouraged to buy and use more than we would were we part of a larger support community; we are urged, in short, to be good consumers. If consumption fails to keep us entertained, we are prodded to reproduce like heterosexuals, i.e., to "have" our "own" biological children through artificial insemination, in vitro fertilization, or surrogacy. If one of us makes more money than the other, we are told that it is acceptable to become dependent on that greater income and follow the moves that accompany a promising career, even if we're half of the relationship—the half that doesn't make the money and stays home with the kids. Gay people today have become experts at impersonating straight nuclear families.

Edmund White

Over the course of the last twenty centuries, intellectuals involved in theorizing Christian morality have set parameters for the role and function of sexual intercourse in the Christian life. From the early admonitions of patristic fathers like Augustine and

John Chrysostom, through medieval moralists such as Aquinas, to
the more recent proclamations of Protestants and Catholics alike,
Christian ethicists and moral theologians have agreed that for sex to
be moral it must involve two ends: unity and procreativity. In recent
history, for example, Pope Paul VI's 1968 declaration in the encyclical *Humanae Vitae*, that "the conjugal act of true mutual love [is
constituted by] unitive and procreative meanings,"[1] is virtually
indistinguishable from Protestant ethicist Paul Ramsey's claim that
"sexual intercourse has two goods or intrinsic ends [which are] its
relational or unitive and its procreative purpose."[2] Although dis-
agreement over the precise meaning and order of these two ends
exists, the community of faith has consistently affirmed that human
sexuality must be both unitive and procreative to be morally acceptable within the Christian paradigm.

Over the course of the last two decades, an unprecedented number of works have attempted to defend homosexuality within the
Christian framework. Because the traditional emphasis on procreativity has often been used by religious conservatives to condemn
homosexual acts (since these conservatives believe that gay people
cannot have children), many of these books have simply side-
stepped the traditional moral logic by arguing for the acceptance of
gays for reasons unrelated to either unitivity or procreativity.
Themes such as the goodness of the human embodiment,[3] the theological power of erotic love,[4] the special spiritual attributes of gay
people,[5] the empathetic and political character of Christ,[6] and the
presence of gay people in the Bible or in Christian history[7] have
grounded theses suggesting that gay people ought to be allowed
full-fledged membership in the Christian Church. The increasing
popularity of these books, along with the growing visibility of progressive Christians on the issue of homosexuality, is changing the
sexual character of many Christian denominations and churches.

In this new wave of gay-affirming scholarship, several works
stand out because they attempt to embrace homosexuality using
tools traditionally associated with the discipline of theological ethics. One significant strand of moral inquiry, for example, uses
Roman Catholic proportionalist reasoning to argue that although
heterosexual unitivity and procreativity are the ultimate goods of
sexual intercourse, stable and monogamous homosexual unions that

at least provide the unitive end are better than unstable, promiscuous sexual practices that might otherwise result. Moral theologians Philip Keane and Vincent Genovesi, SJ, argue that if the option of the celibate life is not available to some homosexuals, it is better for those homosexuals to be involved in loving, monogamous relationships rather than promiscuous, lascivious sexual encounters.[8] Thus, in these works, certain monogamous homosexual unions can be understood as moral, not because they are in themselves good, but rather because they are better than the alternative.*

Another Christian justification of homosexuality rests on the idea that homosexual activity is no less moral than intentionally nonprocreative heterosexual activity; that is, *homosexuality is morally equivalent to the use of birth control.* In this reasoning, both of these practices can be understood as procreative, in a wider sense, as a pledge or assurance that if a new life were to be brought to the relationship, then both partners would welcome and support it together.** Thus, for example, Patricia Beattie Jung and Ralph

---

*Conservative critics of proportionalism would formulate the logic of proportionalism slightly different by arguing that the committed relationship was the "lesser of two evils," and thus suggest that the proportionalists in fact sanction evil. Proportionalists would argue that the endorsement of committed, monogamous relationships is not an evil but a good because it carries with it the partial good of unitivity and avoids the evil of promiscuity and licentiousness.

It is also interesting to note that the proportionalist methodology relies on a rather recent development in the history of sexuality, i.e., that some people possess a "homosexual identity" that stands apart from practice, and that gay people exist prior to and independent of sexual encounters. Thus, these texts do not suggest that gay people should make an attempt to go straight. Rather, they reason that if gay persons cannot be celibate, they ought to be in permanent loving relationships in order to avoid greater sins associated with promiscuity. The idea of a fixed homosexual identity that operates independent of sexual practice is challenged by many contemporary theories.

**Paul Ramsey was the first to develop this interpretation of procreativity as a justification for birth control. He writes that "a married couple engaging in contraceptive sexual intercourse do not separate the sphere or realm of their personal love from the sphere or realm of their procreation, nor do they distinguish between the person with whom the bond of love is nourished and the person with whom procreation may be brought into exercise." Thus, Ramsey argued that birth control is acceptable as long as the people engaging in sexual activity had agreed to be monogamous, i.e., not to procreate with others. Paul Ramsey. *One Flesh: A Christian View of Sex Within, Outside, and Before Marriage.* Nottingham: Grove Books, 1975, p. 4.

Smith argue in *Heterosexism: An Ethical Challenge* that the interdicts against homosexuality, based on procreation, are not successful because "we [Christians] do not consider heterosexual couples who marry but remain childless less married than others who procreate,"[9] and further because "homosexual couples can procreate with the assistance of a third party."[10] Jung and Smith argue that committed, monogamous, same-sex relationships can be as moral as heterosexual unions. Indeed, they argue that discriminatory attitudes toward same-sex unions are the result of the sin of "heterosexism"; Jung and Smith call us to examine and correct not homosexuality, but rather heterosexist bias within the Church today.

It is interesting to note that in each of these texts, *support of same-sex activity is made possible by a condemnation of all sex outside of committed, monogamous relationships.* For the proportionalists, homosexuality inside a monogamous relationship is endorsed precisely so that homosexuals will not be forced to act out their sexual desires in secretive, promiscuous, noncommitted settings; i.e., a committed gay relationship achieves the good of unity while avoiding the evil of promiscuity and licentiousness. For Jung and Smith, the ends of unitivity and procreativity—whether gay or straight—can only happen in committed, monogamous relationships "[b]ecause all human beings must learn how to love each other [and] such schooling takes time, effort and patience. . . Fidelity understood as permanence is a practical requirement necessitated by our need to learn how to love one another."[11] For Jung and Smith, promiscuity is immoral "not because it breaks a specific promise, but because," they argue, "everyone is short changed in the process."

The position that accepts homosexuality only in the case of committed, monogamous relationships is not at all unique to these moralists. On popular levels, Bishop John Shelby Spong, for example, tells us that "[t]he relationship in which sex is shared needs to be exclusive. . . Multiple sex partners at the same time is a violation of vulnerability, commitment, honesty, and the reality of caring."[12] Similarly, Sidney Callahan supports monogamy as the only moral option because, as she puts it, "two persons can become united as one in a way that is impossible for three or four persons." "The symmetry of a monogamous dyad," she explains, "works toward the equality of those in the relationship because there must be constant give and take in a bounded unit, particularly if it continues over time."[13] Indeed, when gay people today seek refuge in Reconciling, Open and Affirming, and More Light congregations,[14] the Church expects them to be either single (and presumably celibate), or involved in a monogamous and permanent relationship. The most progressive of our churches today will bless a same-sex union in a noncivil ceremony, and thus reinforce the idea that it is acceptable to be gay only inside an exclusive relationship.*

This emphasis on monogamy, I suggest, urges gays to mimic heterosexual relational structures. We are told that on the deepest level our allegiance and commitment belong not to our larger community but to our partner or nuclear family. We are encouraged to participate in the American dream by buying a house and living "together," i.e., to separate ourselves from larger kinship systems. While living in this nuclear unit, we are encouraged to buy and use more than we would were we part of a larger support community; we are urged, in short, to be good consumers. If consumption fails to keep us entertained, we are prodded to reproduce like heterosexuals, i.e., to "have" our "own" biological children through artificial insemination, in vitro fertilization, or surrogacy. If one of us makes more money than the other, we are told that it is acceptable to become dependent on that greater income and follow the moves that accompany a promising career, even if we're half of the relationship—the half that doesn't make the money and stays home with

---

*Several exceptions attempt to support nonmonogamous relationships by suggesting that although nonmonogamy is difficult to execute in daily life, it should not be prohibited abstractly. Works by ethicists J. Michael Clark, Carter Heyward, James Nelson, and Mary Hunt do not endorse monogamy as a good end in itself, but rather as a means to the good of a faithful relationship. As Clark represents it, monogamy is "a pragmatic and mutually chosen means for nurturing the most healthy and wholistic sexuality-in-relation for two people committed to a common process of growth and liberation together." (J. Michael Clark, "Men's Studies, Feminist Theology, Gay Male Spirituality" in *Sexuality and the Sacred: Sources for Theological Reflection,* James Nelson and Sandra Logfellow, [eds.], [Louisville: Westminster, 1994] p. 227). Thus, although these ethicists entertain the possibility that a person can sustain more than one loving relationship in theory, I contend that their model for the ideal relationship in practice remains nuclear, isolated, and heterosexual.

the kids. Gay people today have become experts at impersonating straight nuclear families; the only difference is that one of us is the "wrong" gender.

This way of organizing social life is certainly not the only one, and when viewed with feminist and materialist concerns in mind, it is perhaps not even the most moral. Certainly the Christian Church, itself, has had a long history of challenging us to live more connected lives. From St. Benedict to Dorothy Day, from the Anabaptists to the Oneida experiment to the Shakers, the tradition challenges commitments that take primacy over Christian community, including our allegiances to our families. Historically, the Church has attempted to break down the boundaries that exist around primary, particular relationships in favor of relationships and dependencies on a community of believers. Christians throughout the centuries have understood that life in Christ means being responsible to and for many more people than one's spouse and children. Life in Christ, in the most radical sense, demands an openness to other community members. When rightly understood, I suggest that the sexual culture that many gay men have promulgated challenges the hegemony of the nuclear family in a similar manner.

In his *The Culture of Desire*, Frank Browning reports that "by the spring of 1991, New York, Los Angeles, and San Francisco had seen the proliferation of the revived sexual underground. . . . open rooms in the warehouses of depleted industrial zones [appeared], where in the small hours of the morning, young men lined up with their buddies to probe, caress, and gnaw at one another's flesh in dimly lit tangles of animal abandon."[15] These activities, often described as "anonymous," "promiscuous," or "nonrelational" sex, have been criticized as immature or immoral by most factions of American culture, including most liberal-minded Christians. These practices are seen as the product of a particular kind of masculine psychology, which is driven by a base and insatiable sexual desire and which consequently cannot commit to "the real thing," i.e., to a monogamous relationship. I suggest to the contrary that it is worth considering the extent to which gay communities are composed not of men who have failed to meet the "universal" and "self-evident" standard of exclusive relationship, but rather of men who have organized their sexual-social lives on a different model, a model that is fundamentally communal. In these worlds, allegiance to the entire community is often more vital and meaningful than any particular coupling within that community. As Edmund White describes it, "sex has for a long time now been the essential glue holding the urban gay community together."[16] Perhaps what happens in many gay male cultures is not anonymous, promiscuous, or nonrelational, but communal. Indeed, I argue that this communal sense of sex is not at all dissimilar to or incompatible with the Christian tradition's formulation of unitivity. A close examination of both concepts will flesh out the similarities.

In the Christian tradition, the abstract claim of unitivity evokes analogies of intimacy, steadfastness, and one-fleshness. In the unitive nature of the sex act, two are made one. The boundaries of either individual are blurred—both literally and metaphorically—such that each individual becomes, at least momentarily, a part of something larger than himself or herself. As Vincent Genovesi, SJ, describes it, "sexual intercourse is a sign of total, unreserved giving of self. [During sex], the individual's personality is lost in an interpenetration of the other self."* In the act of sex, people are changed for having been merged with the body and spirit of another.

Although all sex acts must produce this unitivity to be moral within the Christian tradition, the unitivity that disrupts our isolation and individualism is not at all confined to one monogamous sexual partner. Indeed, we are called over and over by sacred texts to surrender our individualistic selves to become part of the body of Christ, to be unified with all other Christians into one organism. We are called to love each in Christ even if that love costs us our lives. As Philip Turner states it,

> In Christ, Christians believe that it is no longer necessary to marry in order to escape loneliness. Baptism into Christ pro-

---

*Vincent J. Genovesi, SJ. *In Pursuit of Love: Catholic Morality and Human Sexuality.* Collegeville, Minnesota: The Liturgical Press, 1987, p. 154. Genovesi's work locates unitivity almost completely in the "interpenetration of the moment of orgasm." I disagree with this assertion and believe that orgasm is one of many sexual practices that may or may not produce unitivity. The act of sex, for me then, cannot be defined essentially or fully before the event; indeed, what counts as sex depends on how actions and events are understood and narrated.

vides what was once provided only by marriage, and it is partly for this reason that the early Christians took the unprecedented step of saying that the single state was as honorable as the married one and perhaps even preferable. Once baptized, each person is given both family and friends in such a way that the terrible problem of human loneliness is overcome by incorporation into God's family.*

Thus, the body of Christ is made possible only when we are able to transcend the boundaries of our own selves to become something larger, something part of God. Commitment to another, the tradition teaches us, is always more forceful when you feel that part of yourself lives in the other. Indeed, Rowan Williams goes so far as to suggest that unity is not simply a matter of wanting to be part of another. It is also the feeling of having others want to be part of us, merging the wanter and the wanted. As he puts it, it "is a transformation that depends in large part on knowing yourself to be seen in a certain way: as significant, as wanted."** Unitivity then is not simply an ethereal merging, it is the feeling we get when we are wanted and loved, when we have the good fortune to belong somewhere. "We are pleased," Williams claims, "because we are pleasing."

The excellent works of fiction, memoir, and academic study stemming from and/or commenting on gay urban culture over and over replay the scene where the young man finds his first sex in a bathroom or bar and emerges from that space changed.[17] Each sexual encounter after that shores up his membership in the community he finds there, and his participation and contribution subsequently make the community he finds stronger for others. His iden-

*Philip Turner. "Limited Engagements," in *Men and Women: Sexual Ethics in Turbulent Times*, Philip Turner (Ed.) (Cambridge: Cowley, 1989), pp. 81–82. It should be noted that Turner's work is explicitly condemnatory of homosexual activity; in citing him in this essay, I do not intend to endorse his entire ethical project but only to suggest that his thinking on unitivity is helpful in thinking through issues associated with sexual morality.

**Rowan Williams. "The Body's Grace," Michael Harding Memorial Address, Oxford University, July 2, 1989. (Published by LGCM, 1989, p. 3.) Williams' essay centers around concepts of faithfulness in the realm of sexual desire. While most of his readers assume that such faithfulness can only exist in monogamous relationships, this essay is attempting to explore the possibility that faithfulness can be (and indeed is) operative on a larger, communal model.

tity begins to be defined by the people he meets in those spaces. Although he may not know the names of each of his sex partners, each encounter resignifies his belonging. And although no two members of the community make steadfast promises to any one person in the community, each in his own way promises himself as part of this world. Intimacy and faithfulness in sex are played out on the community rather than individual level. A form of the unitivity described in the Christian tradition is apparent in the cultures and communities that many gay men inhabit.

I suggest, then, that most descriptions of these sexual communities are thus inaccurate. Sex in these worlds is not anonymous, since anonymity implies that the partner is somehow unknown, and as one gay male friend put it, "Even though I may not know his name, I know what music he listens to, what food he likes, where he vacations. His name is incidental. He's part of our world; that's all I need to know." Similarly, sex in these enclaves is far from promiscuous or indiscriminate since partners are chosen precisely because they belong inside that community, and because they show physical signs (such as taste in clothes, food, music) of participating in that world.* Finally, sex in these communities is completely relational because it functions as a way of inscribing members into an identity larger than the individual.

The sex that produces unitivity also produces a desire to be open, to include others. Once we feel the joy that accompanies the breaking down of our own spiritual and physical boundaries, we are able to feel more open about the prospect of sharing new life with and in others. Once the bonds of individualism are broken, we desire to bring others in. We may do so by conceiving children, or by understanding the new life in the union, itself, to be the thing that has been created. As James Hanigan cautions,

> The new life and love to be created and to be shared in [a moral sexual relationship] must not be understood in the first place as the new child to be and the parental love extended to

---

*Indeed, in many communities, the sex itself functions as the first sign of membership; after sex, full-fledged members subsequently school younger members on matters of style and taste to help them identify themselves and each other in greater detail.

him or her. Rather, this new life and new love must first be seen as the new common life and love of the married couple themselves, which in Christian understanding is but their participation in the divine love-life.[18]

Thus, procreative sex has come to mean (within the parameters of most moral theologians*) sex that creates a good relationship and an environment where the newcomer can be welcomed. In this respect, homosexuality that is unitive is no less procreative than unitive heterosexual intercourse that uses birth control. In both instances, new life—something bigger than the sum of its parts—can be formed. In the face of today's reproductive technologies, we must acknowledge that an ethic based on biological reproduction as the sole interpretation of procreativity is inadequate. As Williams states it, "if we are looking for a sexual ethic that can be seriously informed by the Bible, there is a good deal to steer us away from assuming that reproductive sex is a norm."[19] Our focus has shifted from reproduction to creating new life in Christ.

In America today, dozens of young men leave the small towns and heartlands every day and make their way to urban centers because they believe that a community awaits them there. Sometimes they come after reading about Castro Street in a magazine they found left in a bathroom; other times they come having memorized the entire map of New York City, knowing where every gay bar is on that map. Often they are innocent young men who are driven by a desire to find a world where they will be accepted and honored, where they can belong without hiding a part of themselves, where *their* dreams, too, can come true. When they get there, they will find a community of men who will remember what it is like to be young, alone, scared, and broke. They will find men who believe, as Paul Monette writes, that "it's a kind of duty to the tribe to take care of [these kids] and make it all less frightening."[20] They will be initiated into the social fabric of that community not only

---

*That is, Protestant theologians and Roman Catholics who fall outside the official magisterium teaching on the issue endorse this interpretation. My assumption is that there is a general consensus among many Christians that "procreativity" signifies many practices that include but are not limited to human biological reproduction.

through sex but also through crash courses in taste and style. There they will learn to renarrate their lives in the frame of homosexuality, i.e., to recognize many of the things they enjoyed before as simply a prelude to coming out. They will take up residence inside the souls of other men and feel responsible even (and perhaps especially) for those friends with whom they have not shared sex, for they recognize in this community that each is part of the other.

This new culture they inhabit often challenges their own racial or class prejudices. As Browning put it, "[T]he parks and the bathhouses have been places of freedom and fraternity . . . places where the cares and duties of the day dissolved, where barriers of class and education might temporarily evaporate."[21] There is a sense in which the men in the parks, bathrooms, and bars have no separate identity, no history, and no background, except that of belonging to this community. Everything else about them, where they come from, what they do, is eclipsed by their identity as gay men. Moreover, it is important to remember that our gay communities function and grow even in the AIDS crisis. The virus threatens every young man that gets off a bus; everyone who goes to a bar or back room to share sex is potentially vulnerable. Yet they continue to come. They leave behind high school diplomas, families who love them, college educations, chances of advancement, all to be part of this world. AIDS hasn't stopped these communities; indeed, it has only made them stronger.

Some gay men would disagree with my ethical analysis and evaluation. For them, these populations, which I read as community-based kinship support systems, function as locations of adolescent, male, sexual acting out, and as places where one goes only to avoid intimacy and unitivity. J. Michael Clark, for example, argues that these communities "institutionalized patterns of behavior that prevented. . . any possibility of intimacy." He continues,

"Glory holes," which revealed not persons but only penises, utterly blocked relational intimacy; darkened, music-filled bathhouses and orgy rooms likewise presented only vague bodily forms in fog and steam, while they precluded intimate communication and reduced the human participants again to merely genital machines; even the seemingly more personal one-night stands with bargoing "tricks" were generally begun under the veil of dim lights, loud music, and alcoholic haze, consummated often enough without so much as an exchange of names, and, after orgasm, cleaned up and cleaned out of one's life as quickly as possible, lest the postcoital awkwardness give way . . . to any undesired intimacy.[22]

Many others agree with Clark by pointing out the down sides to these worlds, such as the fact that monogamous, permanent relationships are less likely to be sought out because sex is so readily available elsewhere. These critiques ought to be taken seriously because they help us remember that all urban gay communities do not function in the utopian fashion I have outlined here. From my vantage point outside the gay male community, the model of communal sex that operates in many places appears to be based on agreements about the organization of social and sexual life whereby each individual feels himself to be part of the larger whole. Sex in this instance signifies participation in a world where all members are valued and receive love not from one but many. Critics such as Larry Kramer and Andrew Holleran help me remember that many communities are grounded in a landscape where lying, cheating, and adultery are normative; where men make monogamous commitments and break them; where promiscuity is simply a way of avoiding intimacy with one's partner.* Sex in these instances, they remind me, is neither communal nor unitive. Indeed, under such circumstances, sexual violence; humiliation; rape; and discrimination based on race, class, body size, and type are often hard to avoid.** However, rather than proscribe gay communal sex, I sug-

---

*I recognize that in reality, the difference between these two patterns may not always be clear. For example, one partner of a monogamous couple might want to renegotiate the terms of their relationship in order to participate in such a community. We need to think about the differences between what I have called communal sex and those immoral practices signified by words like "lying" and "cheating." In my opinion, this distinction cannot rest on something like consent, as all too often in sexual matters, desperate people agree to situations that they later find untenable.

**Gay communities often have an idea of what "gay" should look like, and those who don't fit the mold are often abused or rejected. We need to learn how to take better care of each other by examining the exclusionary function of our politics and aesthetics.

gest that we use these criticisms of gay culture to identify ways in which our communities could be improved.

Although it is true that not all gay sex is communal or unitive, it is also true that not all heterosexual, monogamous sex is unitive either. In both circumstances, sex can be surrounded by boredom or distraction, and sex can make us close off and feel distant and divergent from the other, rather than part of her or him. Sex can be used to demonstrate one person's power over another. Sex can be a way of keeping our sex partner's spirit from entering our soul. Those immoralities, however, are found just as readily in straight sex as they are in gay male cultures. Monogamy can be a good thing, but it can also be a prison of abuse as well. Communal sex can be a way to exploit each other sexually, or it can be a way of expressing communion with others. Stated simply, monogamy is not a way of ensuring morality. Indeed, my point is precisely that it is incidental to unitive sexuality. The moral nature of the sex act comes only in the context of commitments and associations, in which the act is situated.

Moreover, when a gay community is functioning as a unitive assemblage, it works to teach young initiates how to avoid those people and practices that can hurt them. As part of the function of procreativity, good gay communities teach new initiates how to have "safe sex," i.e., how to protect themselves not only against AIDS but also against persecution and humiliation. Gay fiction and film offer further instructions on how to negotiate safely through the bars and bathrooms, and older gay men take on the role of mentor in helping younger ones find their way in the community. As Armistead Maupin articulates it about his own coming of age, "I learned [from that community] that you could tell the difference between a nice guy and a bastard in the dark."[23]

I believe it is important to investigate the positive, communal aspects of gay culture because these communities are one of the few remaining places where the hegemony of heterosexist, capitalist, patriarchal, nuclear family is challenged. To reproduce the structure of that family with same-sex couples is to reproduce a system founded on their oppression.[24] The Church needs gay communities because Christians have forgotten how to think about social and sexual life outside the family. In the Christian Church in America today, no one needs to risk job, education, family, or health to go to church. Being part of a church is socially acceptable; No one is dying—literally or figuratively—to join. Membership entails no risks, and consequently we don't depend on the support of other parishioners in a way that makes us part of them. We remain separate, individuated Christians, tearing down the walls of our selves only with our husband or wife, only within the fortress of the family, only with one, monogamous other. *Indeed, the "family" has become the master issue for the Christian right precisely because those Christians have totally lost their ability to be dependent and interconnected, because they have lost their ability to be Church.*

Gay male communal sex could function as a model for Christians, then, in two senses. First, Christians could see the gay model of community as a challenge to the isolation that pervades society today, an isolation that is all too familiar in our churches. The hegemony of the nuclear family renders those living outside this structure "alone"; even within the families, loneliness abounds. We are not living as Christians when such isolation occurs. Indeed, as Turner notes, "An issue far deeper than sexual ethics confronts us. It is the absence of a community of Christians in which no one need be alone. The deep issue is not sex but the constitution of the church."[25] Gay men can teach us how to be responsible to a community wider than just our partner and children. The communal lifestyle that our brothers invent shows us how to become a deeper part of one another's lives. Second, we Christians could capitalize on the passion of gay communities by using gay issues to strengthen our own ranks. Many of our denominations are in the unique position at the close of the twentieth century to join forces with gay communities in their struggle to end AIDS and homophobia. Our churches are once again called to take a position to end oppression. But it will cost us. We will lose membership, our houses will be divided, it might even become dangerous for us to attend worship. But, it is this kind of church—one that dares to take prophetic stands in the face of hatred and discrimination—that most of us long for.

I want to conclude by suggesting that the reverse is also true, that we gay Christians need the Church, along with its heretofore homophobic tradition of moral inquiry, to think clearly about the role of sexuality in our lives. Our liberal-based secular supporters prompt us to see the issues associated with homosexuality in church as issues of privacy. Straight Christians ought to be tolerant of our sexual practices, they tell us, because what we do at home is simply a matter of privacy. This strategy feels wrong inside a church that challenges the distinction between the public and private, between the personal and the political. As Christians, we are called to reveal ourselves to one another in order to become part of one another, in order—finally—to participate in the body of Christ. We want a church that offers guidelines for thinking about when sex is good and when it's bad and then celebrates with us and for us when we create and sustain sexual relationships that follow those moral parameters. The Christian tradition gives us a way to understand our gay lives and gay sex as good, not as something that needs to be sequestered into private space.

On the other side, supporters affiliated with Queer studies prompt us to liberate ourselves by denying the necessity of ethical impositions. All sex, they tell us, is good sex. The very idea that sex ought to be a spiritual experience is, for them, limiting and oppressive.* While these works have shed a great deal of light on many gay issues, the agenda they advocate is—on this point—irreconcilable with the Christian tradition. As Jung and Smith note, "Christians have wisely taught that we cannot survive in a community where individual desire is the only criterion for appropriate behavior."[26] We Christians live in a world where sexuality has come to signify

---

*See, for example, JoAnne Loulan's work, which claims, "[We] trap ourselves with shoulds. Sex should be sacred. Sex should be a spiritual union between two people. I don't know about you, but I have done some things during sex that are not all that sacred, and I wouldn't particularly say my spirit was unified with the other woman. I got off." (Quoted in Arlene Stein [ed.], "The Year of the Lustful Lesbian," in *Sisters, Sexperts, Queers* [New York: Penguin, 1993], p. 25.)

At other moments, queer theorists often seem to advocate something that, in my opinion, is not far from unitivity. In her seminal queer work "Thinking Sex," Gayle Rubin suggests, "[A] democratic morality should judge sexual acts by the way partners treat one another, the level of mutual consideration, the presence or absence of coercion, and the quality and quantity of the pleasures they provide." ("Thinking Sex," in *Pleasure and Danger*, Carol Vance [ed.] [New York: Routledge, 1984], p. 283.) It is my hope that Christians could dialogue with queer theorists on the point of whether or not such criteria constitute unitivity.

unitivity, and where discussions about morality surround sex in an attempt to ensure that unitivity. I believe that our task as gay Christians is not to deny that association, but to find ways to fit within it. Stated clearly, the connection between sex and unitivity is a good way for Christians—both gay and straight—to measure the worth and value of their sexual encounters.

Let me be clear that I am not claiming that the connection between sex (gay or straight) and unitivity/procreativity is in any way "natural," but rather that the Christian tradition has constructed moral sex as involving these ends. Those of us who call ourselves Christians live in a world where sex has come to mean something not unlike "holy communion." Although the idea that sex has this meaning has been used under patriarchal and homophobic regimes to limit and regulate sexual behavior, abandoning traditional associations is not the right solution for us. Instead, we must strive to recapture definitions of unitivity and procreativity to encompass those sexual practices that have united us with each other and with God and that we recreate openly and daily for younger generations of gays and lesbians to enter. We are all trying to escape meaninglessness in our lives. We don't want to look back at our ties to other people as a waste of time. We want to escape the hurt that accompanies not belonging anywhere. Some of us do this with people of the same sex, others with opposite-sex persons. Some of us do this by having long-term, monogamous relationships, others by living in communities where love, support, and belonging exist in different patterns. *In any case, the pertinent question is not which partner or pattern is the only ethical one, but rather which kinds of sexual interventions change our lives and make us part of one another, which acts unite us into one body, and which contexts fight meaninglessness.* These questions, which lie at the heart of the moral tradition, ought to constitute the heart of gay activism in the Church as well.

The lines that need to be policed are not the ones between gay or straight or between monogamous and communal, but rather between good and bad sex. We need to talk about what it means to be united in sex; we need to investigate methods of opening ourselves to receive the soul of another; we need to discern what spiritual gifts we need to keep ourselves vulnerable and open to the other; we need to think about when power operates inappropriately or unethically in a sexual encounter. We need to stop worrying about the difference between monogamy and promiscuity and identify what allows sex to be moral and good.

This, of course, won't be easy. Conventional interpretations teach us to make pronouncements on abstract sex acts, for example, sex inside a marriage without birth control is moral, or sex outside marriage is immoral. The boundaries are constructed so that we never have to think about whether or not our own souls are open, desirable, or even wanting. As Williams puts it, "The question of human meaning is not raised, we are not helped to see what part sexuality plays in our learning to become human with one another, to enter the body's grace, because all we need to know is that sexual activity is licensed in one context and in no other."[27] A Christian evaluation of sexuality will return to the heart of the moral tradition by examining concrete practices in context rather than accepting hollow dictums on abstract acts and identities.

To do so today, we must look beyond the issue of blessing of same-sex unions in church into a landscape where the topic of concern is not "homosexual identity" but rather the moral nature of all sexual practices—gay and straight. By allowing the primary issues of gay activism in the church to be ordination and blessing of unions, we obscure the complex sexual lives of many gay people, particularly those who live their lives in more complex communities. In his work on gay sexuality, Williams argues that "same sex relations oblige us to think directly about bodiliness and sexuality in a way that socially and religiously sanctioned heterosexual unions don't."[28] Although I'd like to believe Williams' point, I must note that we still aren't very good at thinking about bodiliness and sexuality clearly. We obstruct our own inquiries about sexual morality, about unitivity and procreativity, with unnecessary dictums about identity and organizational structure. Indeed, in a tradition that has a long and intricate history of discussion around the proper role of sex, the asexuality of gay politics obtrudes in our politics and operates against us.

We can begin to recover the core of the tradition, therefore, by agreeing that communal sex—when it is unitive and procreative—can be understood as legitimate Christian practice that every

Christian could endorse. It is not the only appropriate Christian means of sexual expression, of course, but it is one of many ways that Christians can express commitment, connection, interdependence, unitivity, and procreativity.* When sex acts, whether gay or straight, monogamous or communal, function in ways that lead us to these traditional ends, they ought to be considered moral. It is time that we locate ourselves and the practices we have developed deep in the center of the Church by using ancient norms to judge our behavior.

NOTES

1. Pope Paul VI, *Humanae Vitae: Encyclical Letter on the Regulation of Birth* (Washington, DC: U.S. Catholic Conference, 1968), no. 12.
2. Paul Ramsey, *One Flesh: A Christian View of Sex Within, Outside, and Before Marriage* (Nottingham: Grove Books, 1975), p. 4.
3. See James B. Nelson, *Body Theology* (Louisville, Kentucky: Westminster/John Knox Press, 1992), and James B. Nelson, *Embodiment: An Approach to Sexuality and Christian Theology* (Minneapolis: Augsburg Press, 1978).
4. See Carter Heyward, *Touching Our Strength: The Erotic Power and the Love of God* (San Francisco: Harper and Row, 1989).
5. See J. Michael Clark, *Gay Being, Divine Presence: Essays in Gay Spirituality* (Las Colinas, Texas: Tangelwuld Press, 1987); and Mark Thompson (Ed.), *Gay Spirit: Myth and Meaning* (New York: St. Martin's Press, 1987).
6. See Robert Goss, *Jesus Acted Up: A Gay and Lesbian Manifesto* (San Francisco: Harper and Row, 1993); and John McNeill, *Taking a Chance on God* (Boston: Beacon Press, 1988).
7. See Gary David Comstock, *Gay Theology Without Apology* (Cleveland: Pilgrim Press, 1993), John Boswell, *Christianity, Social Tolerance, and Homosexuality* (Chicago: University of Chicago Press, 1980); and Robert Goss, *Jesus ACTED UP: A Gay and Lesbian Manifesto* (San Francisco: Harper and Row, 1993).
8. See Philip Keane, S. S., *Sexual Morality: A Catholic Perspective* (New York: Paulist Press, 1977); and Vincent J. Genovesi, SJ, *In Pursuit of Love: Catholic Morality and Human Sexuality* (Collegeville, Minnesota: The Liturgical Press, 1987).

---

*I do not mean to suggest that gay men who practice communal sex are—by virtue of that practice—Christian, but rather that a lifestyle based on caring for others in a community is not at all antithetical to the Christian call. That is to say, communal sex between gay men is moral when it is unitive and procreative; this morality, however, doesn't make it Christian, as the Christian life requires more from a person than adherence to a particular sexual code.

9. Patricia Beattie Jung and Ralph Smith, *Heterosexism: An Ethical Challenge* (State University of New York Press, 1993), p. 146.

10. Patricia Beattie Jung and Ralph Smith, p. 218. As Jung and Smith explain,

[F]or gay men a surrogate mother is needed for artificial insemination with the sperm from one or both of the male partners in the union. For a lesbian couple either or both of the parents can have a child with artificial insemination. These ways of providing children in same-sex union, unlike adoption, link one partner in the union to the child biologically . . . Surrogacy is certainly not solely the consequence of modern medicine. The biblical witness on marriage indicates that when wives were infertile other women could and did provide children. The story of Abraham, Sarah, and Hagar is the classic example.

11. Patricia Beattie Jung and Ralph Smith, p. 183.

12. John Shelby Spong. *Living in Sin: A Bishop Rethinks Human Sexuality* (San Francisco: Harper, 1988), p. 216.

13. Sidney Callahan. "Two by Two: The Case for Monogamy," in *Commonwealth,* July 15, 1994, p. 7.

14. These titles represent wings of mainline denominations of gay-affirming organizations (United Methodist, United Church of Christ, and Presbyterian respectively).

15. Frank Browning. *The Culture of Desire: Paradox and Perversity in Gay Lives Today* (New York, Crown Publishers, 1993), pp. 77–78.

16. Edmund White. *States of Desire*, New York: Plume, 1991, p. xiii.

17. As sociologist Steven Seidman reports it in *Romantic Longings: Love in America, 1930-1980* (New York: Routledge, 1991), p. 186 for example,

. . . casual sex [is] viewed as a primary community building force in gay life. Through casual sex, gay men were said to experience heightened feelings of brotherhood and male solidarity . . . Barriers of age, class, education and sometimes race were said to be weakened as individuals circulated in this system of sexual exchange; competition and rivalry between men might give ways to bonds of affection and kinship.

18. James Hanigan. *Homosexuality: The Test-Case for Christian Ethics* (New York: Paulist Press, 1988), p. 90.

19. Rowan Williams. "The Body's Grace," Michael Harding Memorial Address, Oxford University, July 2, 1989. (Published by LGCM, 1989), p. 8.

20. Paul Monette. *Becoming a Man: Half a Life Story* (San Francisco, Harper, 1992), p. 274.

21. Frank Browning. *The Culture of Desire: Paradox and Perversity in Gay Lives Today* (New York: Crown Publishers, 1993), pp. 80–81.

22. J. Michael Clark. "Men's Studies, Feminist Theology, Gay Male Spirituality," in *Sexuality and the Sacred: Sources for Theological Reflection,* James Nelson and Sandra Logfellow (Eds.) (Louisville: Westminster, 1994), p. 217.

23. Frank Browning, p. 80.

24. For an argument that opposes gay marriage on the basis that those gays who did not marry would be "outlaws among outlaws," see Frank Browning, pp. 152–155.

25. Philip Turner. "Limited Engagements," in *Men and Women: Sexual Ethics in Turbulent Times,* Philip Turner (ed.) (Cambridge: Cowley, 1989), p. 83.

26. Patricia Beattie Jung and Ralph Smith. *Heterosexism: An Ethical Challenge* (State University of New York Press, 1993), p. 103.

27. Rowan Williams. "The Body's Grace," Michael Harding Memorial Address, Oxford University, July 2, 1989. (Published by LGCM, 1989), p. 4.

28. Ibid., p. 7.

Chapter 16

What Will We Teach the Children?

Singing Cow (Sonia-Ivette Roman)

In Wicca, ancestors not only are blood relations but also are people for whom we have had a special affinity. For instance, if you are an artist, perhaps you will feel a special connection with Frida Kahlo or Michaelangelo (both Queers). In Wicca, that person would be considered an ancestor because she or he inspired you to grow as an artist.

I am a Wiccan. For those of you who are wondering what that means, it means I am an adherent of an earth religion that follows the cycles of the seasons and worships a living goddess and god. They are called by many names—Oya, Khonshu, Herne, Astarte, Radha, Cerridwen, and Eris. Though Wicca traces its roots to the pre-Christian religions of Europe, its modern form is rather young. Covens are autonomous, and we have no central ruling body or person. We have no "Bible" to guide us through the maze of marriage and family. In fact, our only real "law" is the Wiccan Rede, which states "an it harm none, do what ye will."*

Because of this, Wicca has never had a real basis to discriminate against Queer people. In the past, some did try. However, there were

---

*This is a rather archaic expression, and it means that we may act as we wish, but it cannot cause another person harm. For instance, Wiccans would interpret speaking ill of someone as against the Rede. Some Wiccans, though of course not all, would interpret love magic directed at a particular person to be against the Rede, because you are manipulating that person's will and depriving them of the joy of "doing what they will." Wiccans also interpret "do what ye will" as a command to let others live as they wish, as long as it is not harmful. By this interpretation, homophobia is wrong, wrong, wrong. Homophobic behavior definitely harms others by attempting to tell them how to live, rather than letting people figure it out for themselves.

simply too many of us starting our own groups and interacting with others. Gay Wiccans refused to be left out. We kept going to pagan gatherings and talking to straight pagans about what we were doing, who we were, and why there was no real theological basis for discrimination. Now, homophobic Wiccans will find themselves very much in the minority and struggling to defend their untenable position to other straight Wiccans. I am proud to say that there is a very large contingent of straight Wiccans who march with me every year at the New York Gay Pride march under the banner "Witches and Pagans for Gay Rights."

Why would Queers choose Wicca? It is because we know that the Goddess loves us fully just as we are. Not in spite of the fact that we are Queers, or even because of it. But simply, she loves us as a divine expression of her love in this world. Also, I think Queers choose Wicca because of the freedom of ritual expression.

My own love of the Goddess was always apparent even before I was Wiccan. Growing up as a Roman Catholic, I was very much involved in the worship of the Virgin Mary and St. Thérèsa of Lisieux. Even though my parents were Catholics of a mystical bent (we had *Santeros* and spiritualists in my family), they were somewhat unhappy with my choice of St. Thérèsa. My mother believed that it was not a good sign. She used to take away my St. Thérèsa prayer cards, saying, "St. Thérèsa never got married! It's not good for a girl to emulate a saint like that!" I was lucky that the nuns always had more cards, and, at an early age, I learned to hide them. It is interesting to note that when the Nigerian slaves came to America and were forced to convert, they syncretized the image of St. Thérèsa with that of the Warrior Goddess Oya. It is believed that this goddess is a lesbian. So maybe I had someone watching over me even back then.

Wicca is a religion that reaffirms our connection with the earth and lovingly helps us to realign ourselves with that natural impulse toward wholeness. Family is a part of that wholeness.

In the Puerto Rican community in which I grew up, Mom and Dad weren't the only family members to whom I had to pay attention. There was *abuelita* (grandmother), *abuelo* (grandfather), and assorted *tias* and *tios* (aunts and uncles). In addition, there were the *comai* and the *compai,* who were not related by blood but whose words were listened to closely in my family. It was comai and compai who organized birthday parties for the children. When the children grew into adolescence, they could count on comai and compai to try and listen objectively to their complaints. Comai and compai were also expected to help out financially in case of serious trouble.

In addition to comai and compai, there was a network of neighbors who would provide emergency baby-sitting and even "foster care" if a single parent had to go into the hospital and had no one else to watch the children. In fact, the first lesbians I ever knew were a butch-femme couple who ran the numbers and did occasional baby-sitting in my neighborhood. I had no idea that they were two women because the butch in the relationship affected the white T-shirt, leather jacket, and ducktail hairdo that were common among Latino men in my neighborhood. Even though they were lesbians, and they were supposed to be "sick," according to the local Catholic church, it didn't stop anyone from trusting them enough to let them baby-sit me or other children. Clearly, they made their contribution to the welfare of the neighborhood—both financially and in "community currency," which is far more valuable.*

---

*What does it cost to catch a cab to the hospital? Well, that can be quantified into dollars and cents. But how much does it cost to call your neighbor at 2:35 a.m. to take you, your nondriving lover, and your son (who has a fever of 102° and is vomiting) to the hospital? It is far more valuable because you cannot put a price on it. Community currency is the general tit-for-tat method of contributing to the community. It means that "I'll baby-sit for you on Saturday, but when I need a lift to the hospital, you're driving!"

Community currency includes a feeling of responsibility toward the people in the community, as well as attention to the physical aspects of keeping the community a nice place to live, such as helping to paint murals at the playground, helping to maintain the community garden, or forming a block patrol. The Lesbian Avengers and the Pink Panthers are perfect examples of groups that contribute to their communities by making sure that queers feel safe walking down the streets of Greenwich Village.

Wiccans see the earth as their community and as the living, corporeal embodiment of the Mother. As such, the Wiccan concept of community currency extends to environmental activism. Many Wiccans contribute time and money to such organizations as Greenpeace and Earth First. On a local level, many of us are involved in community beautification projects, and we definitely put up a fight when "progress" means cutting down the trees in the children's local playground. When you begin to see trees, rivers, and the sky as a "body," and, more personally, as the Goddess's body, you feel very protective of her. In preventing the chopping down of trees in our neighborhoods, we serve not only the Goddess but also the community.

When I was growing up, people who kept to themselves and didn't participate in the community were considered stuck-up. To these people, our humble neighborhood was but a pit stop on the way to a two-family house in the suburbs. Such people would quickly find themselves out of luck when emergencies arose. Given my background, the idea of just Mom, Dad, a boy, and girl is lonely, and, frankly, unrealistic. We need our friends, and we need our family.

I feel that choosing your family is very important. Some of us lost our biological families when we came out of the closet, whether as witches or as Queers. To fill that void, some of us moved to large cities to find others like us. Some of us find our communities via the internet. In one rural western town that I know of, gays and lesbians meet secretly for worship in what looks to be an abandoned store, to avoid the prying eyes of the local fundamentalists.

In my pagan tradition, we invite the spirits of the "mighty ones" to join us during worship. Who are these mighty ones? They are the ancestors who have practiced our earth religion in times past. They are family, and as such, we invite them to join us in ritual and in the joyful sharing of food afterward (OK, it's really a potluck supper!). In Wicca, ancestors not only are blood relations but also are people for whom we have had a special affinity. For instance, if you are an artist, perhaps you will feel a special connection with Frida Kahlo or Michaelangelo (both Queers). In Wicca, that person would be considered an ancestor because she or he inspired you to grow as an artist.

Also in the Wiccan community, you will find wiccanings (a pagan version of a christening), where the whole community obligates itself to paying special attention to an infant's spiritual and material needs. You will find handfastings (marriages) between two women or two men, or among one woman and two men or three men. It is the policy of my church to not discriminate against parties who wish to marry, regardless of gender or number. So there is a lot of creative leeway.

In a recent handfasting of two elder ladies, three separate ceremonies were held. One was held on the East coast, one on the West coast, and one was held at a public gathering. This was done so that all members of our "tribe" could participate, regardless of where they were across the country. Also, let's face it, Wiccans love to party, and as the Goddess has told us, "All acts of love and pleasure are my rituals."

As Queer, spiritual people, I feel that not only are we uniquely qualified to question "the way things are," but also it is our spiritual mandate to do it! It is our birthright as Queers to question the status quo and the meaning of family. None of us had our identities explained neatly and handed to us on a silver platter. We all had to figure out what it meant to be Queer. Did it mean bisexual or gay? Did it mean male or female? Did it mean monogamous or polyamorous? These decisions were crossroads in our development. We take nothing for granted. We do not assume that the straight relatives should have custody or that any one particular parent should automatically get custody.

Because Queers cannot take for granted that the law will protect us, we need to be innovative when forming marriage bonds. We must make durable powers of attorney, as well as other time-consuming legal documents, just to make sure that our possibly homophobic parents don't end up with the house after a partner dies. Although the law presumes that if one parent dies, the other one automatically gets custody, this is not the case with Queer parents. If two gay men adopt a child, and one of the men dies, the child might not go to the surviving parent. Essentially, unless we have made specific arrangements in our wills, a child may be taken away from the parent who loves and has raised him or her. Why must we jump through all of these legal hoops just to enjoy the same rights that straights automatically enjoy right *now,* just by getting married? By bringing these issues to the forefront, the U.S. justice system is forced to look at criteria other than gender, marital status, or sexual orientation when deciding who should have custody in a divorce. Hopefully, the criterion is "What is in the best interest of the child?"

But we know that in real life this is not the case. I know a woman who has just come out. She left her abusive husband and is now living in fear that because she is a lesbian her child will be taken away from her during the fight for custody. Her mother has pleaded with her to go back to the abusive husband so that the child will have a "normal childhood." It is sad that this woman's mother considers an abusive man to be "normal" and that it is better that the child be abused by a hateful, straight father than loved by two lesbian mothers.

Unfortunately, sometimes we internalize this idea that Queer people are unsuited for parenthood. One of my former lovers was convinced that lesbians should not have children because it was an "unhealthy" environment. I asked her if she meant that lesbians were unfit to be mothers. She said that our "lifestyle" was not conducive to raising children and that having only one sex raise the child was "just not right." Obviously, she had internalized her feelings of hatred to the point where she felt that she, and other lesbians, were not fit to be mothers.

I believe that Queer parents have a lot to offer children. As Queers, we grow up in an oppressive society that labels our love as sick, immoral, and, until very recently, a psychiatric condition worthy of hospitalization. As a Wiccan, I cannot tell you how astonished I am when heterosexuals see our love as something unnatural. In a world that glamorizes war and graphic violence, I would think that any expression of love would be welcome. Clearly, hatred of gay people has nothing to do with God or Goddess and a lot to do with privilege and power—who gets it, and who doesn't.

When we Queers reach out to help others in need, whether in Amnesty International, at the local soup kitchen, or at a foster home for gay children, it is not only out of a need to be compassionate but also out of an acute awareness that only comes from having been in a social space that accords us few privileges. However, Queers are also aware that feeling compassionate is not enough. Are there not churches who say they are "compassionate" toward the gay person—loving the sinner but not the sin and then barring us from being actively involved in worship?

No, clearly, compassion toward those who are suffering is not enough. And so, we teach our children to act upon their compassion. I remember one bitter autumn day, I was walking with a friend, her lover, and their daughter. We passed a homeless man, who was clearly very cold. The little girl took off her scarf and said, "Mommy, can I give it to him?" My friend told her she could, and I watched as she cautiously approached and gave him the scarf. What had my friend taught her daughter? That fear is not an excuse for inaction, and we must act to effect change. As Queers, we truly believe that even the smallest actions can make a significant change in the world. As such, we are careful not to reserve our praise only for the most visible leaders in the gay rights movement, but we remember to lavish it on the folks who stuff envelopes at a fund-raiser or clean up afterward. We praise the little actions because they help turn the wheels of change. Sometimes, they lead to bigger actions, and sometimes, lots of little actions pile up and roll on down the mountain like a landslide. We teach our children not to be afraid that their contributions won't be valued, to feel the fear, and do it anyway.

Like Queers, we Wiccans try not only to be tolerant toward people who are different but also to embrace difference as a part of our strength. You will never, I hope, hear a Wiccan say that Wicca is the one true religion. Frankly, we like diversity, and we certainly don't believe that "one God fits all." This idea, that "My religion is the one true religion" has led to the Crusades, the Ottoman Empire, the conquest of the Americas, and the Inquisition. In case you are thinking "Well, that was then. We're so much more civilized, now," think again, friend. The modern list is equally chilling: the persecution of Tibetan Buddhists by the Chinese, the war in Bosnia, and the murder of doctors who perform legal abortions right here in the United States.

It seems to me that one of our missions as Queers in the world is to show people that a diverse community not only can survive but also can thrive. We do this by pooling our unique strengths toward a common goal. This, too, is a tribal characteristic. To survive, members of the tribe had to specialize in different areas. Everyone had her or his specialty, but no one specialty was valued over another. Some knew where to find the best plant foods. Some knew which plants would cure and which would harm. Some knew how best to position a house so that sunlight would filter through correctly. All of these talents were equally important. This value, that our strength lies in our diversity, is one of the best gifts that we can give our children.

By watching us interact with others during the struggle, our children pick up the idea that many different people working together toward a common goal is fun and makes life interesting.

They learn to interact with a wide variety of people. Can you imagine what would have happened to our early ancestors if they had decided that all brown-haired people were the food gatherers? Or that all redheaded people would be the hunters? Quite simply, they would have died out. Early peoples had to be flexible, and they had to stick together to get the job done.

For modern Queers, getting the job done means creating a world in which each of us can live out our lives in joy (which is our Goddess-given right) and creative fruitfulness. We know that we can create this world by hard work and lots of love. Wiccans do not believe in joyless struggle. We know that we can only get the job done by cooperation, and this is another important value that we pass on to our children.

Our years of working as political activists, on all levels, from letter-writing to clinic escort to socially responsible investing, gives us the tools to work with others toward a common goal. We have had to work through our own differences together. We have had to work through our own personal barriers, such as sexism, racism, ageism, and ableism. In our work, we have had to strategize. For example, we had to determine things such as what is the best way to get a particular politician to back a gay rights bill. Would a letter-writing campaign work? Would protests outside her or his office work? Would talking to other politicians work? In hashing these things out, we learn compromise and cooperation, another wonderful value that we teach our children.

As Queers, we are uniquely qualified to question gender stereotypes. Go to any gay pride march and you will see butch men who sew and femmes who do carpentry; women who used to be men, who are now lesbians; and men who used to be women. Even in butch/femme relationships, I have seen butches who had gorgeous flower gardens and femmes who could take apart a bicycle with their eyes closed. Who better than Queer men and women to teach children that they are not bound to do *anything*—cooking, cleaning, household repairs—according to gender.

It warms my heart to see Queer people educating others about gender stereotypes. I remember one family, headed by two gay men, who had a boy who was taking both ballet and karate lessons. Clearly, they wanted him to be able to express himself creatively in realms that are thought to be feminine (ballet) and masculine (karate). *Many Queer Wiccans believe that gender is fluid, and although we may inhabit a male or female body, we feel free to explore.* As such, we teach our children that it is OK to play with whatever toy they like—trucks, dolls, teddy bears, building blocks, or Barbies—regardless of their gender.

Like straight parents, we do our best to provide our children with a safe, happy home. However, as Queers, we offer so much more. We offer a safe place in which to explore ideas about gender. We teach them the value of community and cooperation. We teach them to be compassionate and to act on their compassion. We teach them that biology is not the sole basis of family. And we teach them to love diversity and embrace it as part of their strength.

Chapter 17

Webs of Betrayal, Webs of Blessings

Leng Leroy Lim

My friends gathered. We read a passage from the Bible about how Jacob wrestled with the angel of God. The angel blessed Jacob with the new name "Israel," but not before maiming his hip. My friends now named me, giving me many names that described my relationship to them, names that showed me who I had become. Each new name they gave me awakened a part of me, typing different narratives and pathways, and opened my eyes to see myself ever more fully. Then it was my turn to reclaim Leng for myself. I symbolically laid Leroy, my public name for 30 years, to rest by putting a childhood cross I had worn into a box. Out of that box I pulled a dragon medallion a friend had given me years ago, but which I had been too ashamed to wear. I then renewed my baptismal vows, and in the confession of my faith, I regrounded myself in the love of my God. Taking a blade, I cut a cross over my heart. With the blood I wrote "Dragon" in Chinese characters on a piece of organic rice paper and burned it. Mixing the ashes in a bowl of wine, I drank it. Years ago, my paternal grandmother had brought home blessed papers from the temples and burned them, dissolving the ashes in water for me to drink so that I would be protected from evil spirits. By performing a similar act, I was reclaiming the blessings of my pagan ancestors, which I had been mistakenly made to renounce in my baptism years ago. By marking my body, and drinking my own life, I took into myself all the pain and wonder of my life into myself. I felt the previously unfelt sorrows of the years, and I also felt a power surging from within, awakened by the embodied love of God as found in my family of friends.

This essay is about the stories I learned from my family, culture, and religion—stories that both blessed and wounded me. This is about how I am making a story of my life. Stories give context and content, and the meaning that is extracted from the retelling of a story in turn becomes the real story. From this, we make a set of new decisions and are off on a whole new path, writing the second chapter.

However, I am aware that not all meaning-making, which we extract from the retelling of stories, necessarily sets us toward life-giving journeys of transformation. The Nazis' recasting of the Versailles Peace Treaty as a stab in the back orchestrated by Jews is an example of such retelling and meaning-making where one story (racial purity) annihilated millions of Jews, homosexuals, Gypsies, mentally disabled persons, Jehovah's Witnesses, and other outcasts. In America, the retelling of World War II victories hides the story of the internment of Japanese Americans. When the process of retelling a story serves to silence or hide other dimensions of the larger story, we start on a journey of incoherence, and we lose touch with our common human need to explore multiple layers of meaning and being in living. What becomes important, then, is the defense of a particular version of a story, so that fundamentalism becomes the only meaningful act left.

Family is the story that a few people have decided to make together. Unfortunately, in America today the fundamentalist version of family allows for only one story: that of a male and female coming together to produce children. This version is a rather curious form of biological reductionism—even for heterosexuals—that betrays the obsession with sex of its fundamentalist authors.

I learned from my paternal grandmother that families go beyond mere biology. Born during the last years of the Qing Dynasty in Fukien Province, China, Granny had her feet bound. She never knew her poverty-stricken parents because she was sold to my great-grandmother to nurse. Together, they fled the poverty of a collapsing dynasty by immigrating to Southeast Asia. As a young girl, she bought a baby boy who was being sold on the streets of Singapore. Retelling the story, she said, "I wanted to hold and feed him." He became my *ku kong,* or granduncle. When I asked her in a taped interview who her real mother was, she insisted that greatgrandgranny was her real mother because "She fed me her milk and her saliva.*

---

*Chinese parents test the temperature of hot food by cooling it in their own mouths before feeding the regurgitated food to the child, hence the metaphor of "saliva" for the filial connection.

Who birthed me is another matter." I learned from her that a family is not only about biology, but also about intentionality, care, and choice. Families are stories about our (mis)adventures in relationships.

This is the story of how I came to acquire the name Leng Leroy Lim. It was a cold New England winter on the eve of the Chinese Year of the Dog. Gathered around me were four friends whom I had invited to be part of my naming ritual.

For some years my parents had been telling me to get rid of my Chinese name Leng, which means "dragon." I was born prematurely, and my early arrival prevented my parents from consulting the older relatives for a Chinese name. Thus, they named me after the year of the dragon in which I was born. With its mythical and imperial significance, the dragon is an auspicious Chinese figure. (The phrase "children of the Dragon" means Chinese people.) When my parents became fundamentalist, charismatic Christians— ironically as a result of my becoming a Christian a few years earlier—they came to believe that the dragon was synonymous with the devil. My retort that the dragon in the Bible is a Hellenistic dragon, and therefore not the same entity as the Chinese dragon, did not convince them otherwise.

To be asked to change one's name, especially by the parents who first gave it, is to be repudiated. My parents, however, assured me they were doing this out of love, as if love could sufficiently justify their denunciation of my personhood. But it is no surprise that love can be used to justify abuse, for part of the Christian tradition has used the need to share "gospel love" with unbelievers to justify ethnic extermination, racism, slavery, misogyny, colonialism, heterosexism, and forced conversions. Such love is about power and not about shared life.

In a curious self-betrayal of this knowledge of their own abusive use of love, fundamentalist Christians have projected onto homosexuals what they won't admit about their own duplicity when they claim that homosexual love, even though it is love, does not make homosexuality right. It might be truer to say that fundamentalist Christian love, while passionate, does not make fundamentalism right, Christian, or loving. Not surprisingly, the socially designated pariah (the "homo" in this case) always carries the blame for the crimes the accusers, themselves, commit.

In contrast, the fullness of the biblical tradition tells a story of love that always respects the integrity of the ones being loved. In the Jewish Scriptures, the story is of a frustrated God who demands love and obedience from Israel by threatening punishment. Yet the story shows that God learns that God cannot compel love to be accepted or else divinity would destroy the free-willed humanity God has created. Thus, the disobedience of Israel is met by divine forgiveness again and again, and not by the annihilation that had been promised. In the Christian Scriptures, tradition holds that this God becomes human and walks the path of love by risking betrayal and death to show that true love must embrace the utter integrity of the other who is being loved, even if that one is an enemy. *This Christian love story, which has gathered disparate people into family, says that love converts by hospitality, not hostility.*

My parents' subconscious message in the name change was not lost on me: "There is a part of you, which we have given you, that we think is completely evil, and we want to absolve ourselves of it." Dragon equals gay equals devil. I eventually returned to Singapore after more than a decade in the United States to come out to them. Setting aside a year from Harvard to accompany them through the process, I was met with prayers, laying on of hands, and the casting out of demons. One night, I found myself sleepless, my body racked with incredible pain. At bedtime, they had asked to pray for me "because we love you," and how can a child say no to that? As they prayed for my healing, a fear like I had never felt before since my teenage evangelical Christian days gripped me. "What if my homosexuality is a curse from the devil?" Five years of gay activism and months of therapy went down the drain as I felt myself disintegrating. I was fourteen again, afraid of my passions, and hoping that Father God or Mother Church would rescue me. Now, my previously estranged parents had finally come to the rescue, and we could all be a happy family! Then quietly came a thought: "You are thirty, not fourteen! The pain is not the devil; it's Mom and Dad. You are being possessed by their shit." Getting out of bed, I lighted my sage stick and started cleansing my room. "Take back your shame, guilt, and pain. I no longer carry your load, nor do I accept your prayers. May everything coming from you return to you." I collapsed onto my bed sobbing and exhausted. I had started the first step of divorcing my parents, at least the parents in my psyche and soul. The somatic pains disappeared, and in their place was another pain—an ache in the heart from the freedom that comes with acknowledging loss.

Either the Devouring Parent archetype (represented by Church, culture, Bible, country, and parents) dies in us, or else we commit suicide, as so many gay, lesbian, bisexual, and transgendered youth have literally done. When the oppressive parent in the psyche dies, you are not orphaned. Rather, you grow up and make your own family.

My friends gathered. We read a passage from the Bible about how Jacob wrestled with the angel of God. The angel blessed Jacob with the new name "Israel," but not before maiming his hip. My friends now named me, giving me many names that described my relationship to them, names that showed me who I had become. Each new name awakened a part of me, tying different narratives and pathways, and opened my eyes to see myself ever more fully. Then it was my turn to reclaim Leng for myself. I symbolically laid Leroy, my public name for thirty years, to rest by putting a child-hood cross I had worn into a box. Out of that box I pulled a dragon medallion a friend had given me years ago, but which I had been too ashamed to wear. I then renewed my baptismal vows, and in the confession of my faith, I regrounded myself in the love of my God. Taking a blade, I cut a cross over my heart. With the blood I wrote "Dragon" in Chinese characters on a piece of organic rice paper and burned it. Mixing the ashes in a bowl of wine, I drank it. Years ago, my paternal grandmother brought home some blessed papers from the temples and burned them, dissolving the ashes in water for me to drink so that I would be protected from evil spirits. By performing a similar act, I was reclaiming the blessings of my pagan ancestors, which I had been made to renounce in my baptism years ago. By marking my body, and drinking my own life, I took into myself all the pain and wonder of my life into myself. I felt the previously unfelt sorrows of the years, and I also felt a power surging from within, awakened by the embodied love of God as found in my family of friends. We ended the morning with a Eucharist celebrated by an Episcopal priest friend and then adjourned for a Boston *dim sum* to celebrate the coming New Year.

The reclaiming of my name was an act of recognizing a basic goodness that had come to me at birth, and which had been miraculously bestowed upon me by my parents, however unconscious their intentions had been. Yet many of us Queer folks, in coming out to our parents have had to say at some point, "No, of course it's not your fault; you didn't make me gay." Do we mean to say homosexuality is not a fault, or that it is not an inherited gift? Surely homosexuality becomes a fault only when not received as a gift. All that we are—the fire in the belly and the ache in the bones—come from an unbroken line of millions of years of (heterosexual!) lovemaking. Call this evolution or the genetic code, but also call all this ancestral gift. Call it God. The wonder of heterosexual union is the new, unique yet ancient life form that is born. When Queer people honor their unique selves, they may be the ones who most profoundly honor the family and the wonder of heterosexual intercourse because we recognize the mysterious gifts of the ancestral line. By honoring the name with which my parents had unconsciously blessed me, by honoring the dragon—that binatured creature of water and air that prefigured the divine-human Christ—I had come to honor the foundations of my soul and the God who had laid those foundations.

One of the earliest phrases I learned in grade one of Chinese school was that "a mother's love is the greatest love." My mother's courage, resilience, love, and generosity have been enormous in my life. She held a job as a schoolteacher for twenty-five years while suffering from a debilitating medical condition. For twelve of those years, my father was estranged and absent, and as a single parent, she supported both of us along with her infirm mother and brother. She taught me English, Mandarin, and Hokkien, and imparted to me a sensitivity of soul. One of the earliest stories we learned was that of Mencius,* the most influential Confucian scholar of ancient China. Mencius' mother moved their residences three times to secure for her son a positive moral environment in which to grow. Once, when Mencius left a task unfinished, she taught him about his moral failing by cutting the cloth she had been painstakingly weav-

---

Mencius is the Latinized form of the Chinese name *Meng-tzu.*

ing. Such was her passion, and, reflecting on our own mothers, we wrote essays about the greatness of mother's love, *wei-da de mu-ai*.

A few weeks after my coming out, in the middle of a conversation about the devil having infiltrated my mind, my mother fell on her knees, speaking in tongues. Screaming, she cursed, "In the name of Jesus, may you never have a male lover."*

Snap went the scissors across the many woven strands of our relationship. Mother's love may be the greatest, but it need not be life-giving.

In returning to Asia, I had no illusions about facing Chinese homophobia, derived from the shame at the loss of "face." But I also knew that there was an Asian permissiveness and generosity toward difference, a "live and let live" mentality for dealing with unresolvable conflicts. However, I was unprepared to encounter a virulent and bigoted Christianity that smelled stronger and stronger of odious American fundamentalism and to have that come forth from the mouths of Chinese pastors—and my parents! The connection of American fundamentalists and Southeast Asia is a literal relationship. The local Christian bookstores are filled with tapes and books from fundamentalist right-wing presses in the United States. The local Anglican church had recruited an ex-gay man from Kansas (oh, Dorothy!) to run Exodus, a ministry started in the United States, which claims to convert homosexuals.** According to my parents and their Assembly of God church, homosexuality was evidence of the end times. I realized, however, that apocalyptic Christianity with its millennialism and restorationism were the new colonizing cults from the West.[1] With humiliation, I saw that this religious imperialism, after years of political independence from

---

*At the time, the experience was more unnerving than it was hurtful. Gregory Max Vogt, in *Pathological Christianity*, relates a similar story, in which a husband, facing possible divorce from his wife, commands her in God's name to come back to the house. (Gregory Max Vogt, *Pathological Christianity: The Dangers and Cures of Extremist Fundamentalism*, Cross Cultural Publications, 1995, p. 3.)

**The two founders of Exodus International, Michael Bussee and Gary Cooper, have since become ex-ex-gay after falling in love with each other and coming out for a second time. See the video *One Nation Under God* (Teodoro Maniace and Francine M. Rzeznik, producers; 3Z/Hourglass Productions, 1993), which documents the problems and deceptions of the ex-gay ministry.

white colonialists, had been possible because some Singaporean Christians had colluded in their own religious recolonization.*

So why do I remain a Christian? When I was twelve years old, and one year into puberty, a schoolteacher friend of my mother gave me a small storybook. In it, a young American boy with blond, tousled hair finds the courage to visit an old lady who lived down the street from him—reputed to be a witch by the neighbors. In the denouement, she turns out to be a kindly Christian woman. She asks him if he has ever heard of Jesus and his love. No, *we* hadn't, *we* said. Then she explained that God loved the world so much that God sent his son Jesus to die for our sins and be our friend. Would *we* like to receive Jesus into our hearts? *Both of us* said yes, and there in my little room, in the sultry tropical heat of a Singaporean afternoon, an immense weight of loneliness lifted off my shoulders, and welling up from within me came a surging wave of feelings I could barely control.

I had fallen in love with God. I had also fallen in love with my soul mate, that little vulnerable, courageous, and beautiful boy with the tousled blond hair. As much as I have searched for God through the years, I have searched for that boy who had first shared my experience of love. This was the coming of Christ in my life and body, and my relationship with this mystical source of being would first carry me into a long, painful struggle with the narrow Christian ideology as represented by the publishers of that little book before I could move beyond it.

Two years after this love encounter with Jesus and the boy with tousled hair—a love I was beginning to realize was supposed to be

---

*With the exception of the Philippines and pockets of old Roman Catholicism established by the Portuguese and Spanish, Protestant Christianity is the newest religion in Southeast Asia. In Singapore, the majority of Christian adherents are Chinese converts from the Little Traditions of Taoism, Buddhism, and Confucianism. Although a minority race in the region, Chinese people in the Indo-Malayo region are economically better off, though politically marginal. Singapore is the exception. Chinese people are the dominant race, but they are conscious of the fragility of their political status. This equation of economic prosperity, qualified political confidence, ethnic marginality and dominance, and neophyte devotion makes religious fervor among Chinese Christians (and others who pick up on the tenor) particularly strong. They also mirror the experiences of certainty, racial (white) confidence (though that is always perceived as under siege), sense of political marginality and dominance, and conversion fervor.

incompatible—I found myself at a charismatic rally held on the grounds of the Anglican cathedral in Singapore. All around me people were praying with uplifted arms, and strange sounds were coming out of their mouths. Not knowing what to expect, I stepped forward to be blessed by the visiting English evangelist. Instead I found the bishop in front of me, asking me what I wanted. I found myself saying, "Ask God to make me more loving." (Did I feel unlovable then?) But under my breath I pleaded, "God, don't make me a homosexual."

What happened next was beyond my comprehension as an ecstatic, painful, and utterly pleasurable surge of fire coursed through my body, threatening to turn me inside out. My knees buckled, and I found myself lying on the ground sobbing, speaking incomprehensible sounds, somewhat frightened by the power I had felt, but incredibly loved and held. Later, I was told that I had—in the jargon of the Charismatics—been baptized in the Holy Spirit. The experience first gladdened me because I felt God had made Godself known to me. Later, as my attraction to boys remained unabated, I start to hate myself. Clearly, if God had touched me with his own presence and yet refused to hear my prayer for sexual change, I had to be despicable.

For anyone who has heard coming-out stories, the years of my teenage life would be terribly clichéd, were they not so painful. The sight of a beautiful boy or emotional intimacy with a male friend would delight and terrorize me. Sneaking into the sexuality section of the Christian bookstores, I would furtively search for the chapter on homosexuality, only to find either silence or condemnation. Over and over I returned to find a new book, and each time I found myself reading my own death sentence. The books recommended fasting and prayers, and I had done all that and nothing had changed. Perhaps God didn't require my prayers as much as my life. After all, had not Jesus said to pluck out your eye if you lusted after a woman? Perhaps I should destroy my body for lusting after men? Too cowardly to take my own life, I groveled to please God by becoming more fundamentalist, crusading against my Singaporean classmates who were Muslims, Hindus, and Buddhists for being devil worshippers. I also chastised women for not submitting to men.

I never imagined when I was fourteen years old that my struggle with spirituality and sexuality would take another fourteen years to finally be resolved. At twenty-eight years of age, I found a community of brothers and sisters at the Body Electric School.* Although I had been publicly out of the closet for a few years, I would only now begin to come out inside, healing the internal wounds.

In a retreat house in New Hampshire, I found myself in a spacious wooden room with twenty-five other men, our ages ranging from twenty-eight (me being the youngest) to seventy years. Our bodies told stories of addiction, operations, accidents, age, work, grooming, leisure, and racial heritage. I was witnessing the life cycle of men and for the first time felt myself a part of an unfolding future. I lay down on a massage table and put on a blindfold. A soft tune with a steady drumbeat played in the background. Somewhere the voice of the leader said, "Wake up the body of your sacred brother; be with him in your breath and touch." I took a deep breath, and the sound of a common sigh coursing through the room joined us together as interconnected beings. Two pairs of hands, warm, gentle, and firm touched me on my heart and genitals and I was gently rocked from side to side. "Open your hearts and genitals, say yes to life and love." I shuddered at the words. As the warm oil was spread along the sixth chakra, I found myself drenched in painful sensations of pleasure. Strong hands kneaded my aching muscles, so long untouched—and my aching heart, so long yearning. I took another breath and let out a long moan. The battle for integrity was almost won.

Being gay is like being born with a compass that is orientated east toward the holy sun of a fiery desire. In the early years, you explore the world with this compass, and it is quite wonderful. You realize soon enough that you walk in a world where most people are going in a different direction. So you try using the maps that family,

---

*The Body Electric School was founded in the 1980s by Joseph Kramer, who had once been a Jesuit in training. A variety of traditions are used: tantra, yoga, Taoist traditions of circulating erotic energy, and Native-American chanting. Its purpose is healing touch, including erotic massage. Gay men come to explore alternate ways of being erotic, and, along the way, learn to touch the depths of the psyche and soul. Its current director, Colen Brown, has extended the work to include women. See also Chapter 14 of this volume.

religion, and culture have given you. But the maps are written with a different compass orientation, and your trip, far from getting better, gets much worse. Because you trust those who gave you the maps, you blame yourself for getting lost. Looking for the safe pasture promised by the maps, you eventually find yourself looking down a cliff edge, wishing you were dead.[2]

On two major climbing expeditions in Alaska, I have had to learn to put aside the detailed topographical maps. However well-made, maps at that altitude cannot accurately plot the characteristics of snowdrifts, shifting glaciers, and hidden crevasses, which change from day to day. Maps provide general characteristics, which have to be interpreted with care. Interpreting the stories on the maps, we found ourselves relying on each other, on our individually acquired skills, on our instruments and intuition, and always sharing stories of past experiences on other snowy mountains.

One day, high on the snow-covered shoulder of Mount St. Elias (named after Elijah of the still small voice, I Kings 19:12), which is the world's tallest coastal mountain, I put aside my religious maps. I burned the homophobic and xenophobic parts of the Bible, praying to God thus, "These words once gave life to your people Israel, but they are now used by the enemies of my people to bring death to us. I return these words to you, that your Word may come forth with life again." Psychically, I had broken both the power of Biblical literalism in my life, and the internal instruments that upheld that way of being in my soul.

Biblical literalism, or fundamentalism, has less to do with being faithful to God and more to do with making sure that God and we are on the same side and *the others are not.* Biblical fundamentalism has soothed and secured the Western conscience during five centuries of colonialism, and the method is being adopted by other cultures now, like my own in Singapore.* In the end, religious fundamentalism's only purpose is to make the world safe for those who are on God's side—a rather curious need for safety, given that God is already on their side. But then, if this annihilating God is

---

*The Anglican Bishop of Singapore, whose jurisdiction is the tiny island of Singapore, has made it Singapore's mission to proselytize Vietnam and Cambodia now that these countries are politically less restrictive.

believed to be so ready to destroy everyone else, what reason is there not to believe he wouldn't do the same to his own? In fact, an Oxford-trained theologian and Pentecostal minister in Singapore, whom my parents had dragged me to see, had said to me, "Once saved, not always saved." The devastating spiritual corollary is once loved, not always beloved. Apparently, given my homosexuality, my baptism and personal experiences of Christ did not guarantee me salvation. *So this fundamentalist God demands fundamentalist loyalty, but cannot fundamentally provide security.* What is this but the Mafia Father-God of the missionaries and "evangelical Christians," a God who will shoot the kneecaps off his own children as a way of "testing and loving" them? Unmask, judge, sentence, and banish the Godfather.

As I lay on the massage table at the retreat house, I listened to the voice directing me to "Return to the breath, stay with the present, feel the now." Now it was time to come home, to come home into the present, into myself and into my body. "Brothers, breathe in life. Take twenty breaths and hold. Hold and squeeze." I held the last breath, suspending it, squeezing every muscle in my body until I shook in spasms. I held onto the breath, feeling frustration, then sadness, then desperation, until it seemed I was strangling myself. "Release the breath, brothers. Release." Still I held on, the loss, the rage, and the pain sweeping over me. I had been trampled by my dear mother, culture, and church. "Forgive us our trespasses as we forgive those who trespass against us," whispered a voice from somewhere. I screamed and let go, surrendering.

Then the FIRE surged through me again, fourteen years later. I saw myself back on the cathedral grounds. Like St. Peter who saw a net with unclean animals descending, and God's voice saying "Eat, nothing is unclean" (Acts 10), I saw Siva; Kuan-yin, the boddhisattva of compassion; and a smiling Chinese dragon dancing with Jesus and my old bishop. There is nothing accursed, says the Book of Revelation. I understood why God had not answered the prayer I had made at the age of fourteen; it was not possible for me to be filled with love and not also have much of that holy energy turn toward the souls and bodies of men. I would learn from Carter Heyward, first from her books, and then from our personal friendship, that the erotic life is about sharing in the passion of God.

Why am I still a Christian? Because I am part of the Christ story, *and the love story now writes me.*

Now came the casting of the web. They had come from across the country in answer to my call to build for me a protective web of sustenance on the eve of my ordination as deacon in the Episcopal Church. These men and women had been part of my journey toward healing in the past. I had written them to say that much as I looked forward to my ordination and ministry to the hurting people of Christ's body, I was afraid that a homophobic Church would devour me. Besides, how was I to keep sane working as a leader in a tradition that much of the time has wanted to see me (as a gay Asian man) destroyed or colonized? Worse still, might I betray myself, my gay and lesbian kin, and others God would entrust to me because of my own fears, wounds, and loneliness? Would they come to be my web of lovers?

In the diminishing light of an early Cambridge summer we gathered. We touched, we danced, we breathed, we sang. During one part of the long and incredibly lovely evening, two men, lovers for approximately twenty years, sat me down in the middle of the circle. They brought out a bundle of warm, orange fabric, cut into long strips but joined at one end. They tied the end around my waist, and each one of the gathered tribe took up the loose end so that I was indeed caught within a web. Then one by one they spoke to me. Their words created a mirror that allowed me to see myself in wonderful, grateful, multilayered ways. Looking at them, I realized that what I loved in them was also what I had in me. Their words washed over me, soothing, stinging, stirring. For the first time in my life, I allowed myself to *hear and receive*. For so long, the closet made me fake it. I thought I had been accepted to Princeton and Harvard by mistake. No words of compliment or love could I trust. Now I believed.

Of the many intimate and powerful words branded on my heart, one sentence has stood out, in part because of the profound shadows the words have embodied. He said to me, "I hold this strand, Leng, to tell you that sometimes when you tug at this, I may not be at the end, and you will find there is no one here." *Eli, Eli, la'ma sabachtha'ni*—my God, why have you forsaken me? And looking into this brother's eyes, I saw that this truth, too, is part of the rhythm of love.

Later that evening, a friend made an incision over the cross I had cut on my heart earlier in the naming ceremony. I would own my pain, and I would also know that my Christ, and his body, the community, have held my pain already. In letting go, I found open spaces within to welcome my tribe and my family.

For myself, as a Queer man, the return to and of love is an acknowledgment that home will ultimately not be in the family (biological or otherwise), the Church (however welcoming), nor even in a potential lover or boyfriend. These are at best oases, places and moments to rest and play. Rather, God is the uncontainable true home, and the self is the hearth and the burning fire.

I recall that when I was in kindergarten, my mother dressed me up in an ancient-looking Chinese silk gown (ah, the beginning of drag!) and entered me in a children's fashion show as the young Yüeh Fei, the legendary General of the Sung Dynasty. When Yüeh Fei was a youth, his mother had tattooed on his back the words "Jin Zhong Bao Guo," or "unfailing loyalty to emperor and country." Years later, framed by his Prime Minister, Yüeh Fei was executed by the Emperor. Chinese people have remembered this betrayal by sticking two pieces of leavened dough together (to resemble the Prime Minister and his wife) and deep-frying them. A breakfast staple, these *you tiaos*—a pun on the Minister's name—can be found everywhere, from Beijing to American Chinatowns.

Who really betrayed Yüeh Fei? Could it not have been the Emperor? Certainly, the Tian An Men massacre of 1989 is the most recent in a series of imperial betrayals in the history of the Chinese people. Perhaps it was Mother Culture, whose tattoos and values made Yüeh Fei (and how many of us?) formulaic and unquestioning? Perhaps it was Yüeh Fei, himself, so conditioned to cultural norms that he did not resist? Nevertheless, when Chinese people eat *you tiaos,* they do not think about the betrayal and retributive rage embodied in the greasy fritters. Time has provided for the fritters to simply be an item of sustenance, the cholesterol notwithstanding. Perhaps the question to ask of Yüeh Fei should be how was he sustained? Was it mother's love? Or love of country and people? Or love of the father emperor? Or simply love, loyal and strong?

Loyalty, or *zhong* 忠 , shows the pictograph of a heart 心 that is centered 中 . Certainly, Chinese people through the ages have remembered, loved, and honored Yüeh Fei's story.

NOTES

1. Although Michael Moriarty's treatment rests on his Bible-centered ideology, the description of the New Charismatics' focus on dominion, restoration, and apocalyptism is detailed and comprehensive. Michael G. Moriarty. *The New Charismatics: A Concerned Voice Responds to Dangerous New Trends*, Zondervan, 1992, pp. 87–182.

2. See Leroy Aarons, *Prayers for Bobby: A Mother's Coming to Terms with the Suicide of her Gay Son* (HarperCollins, 1995), which tells the story of how Bobby Griffith jumped off an overpass because the maps betrayed him.

Chapter 18

We Are *Not* Your Hope for the Future
Being an Interracial Lesbian Family
Living in the Present

Mary L. Foulke and Renee L. Hill

We are convinced of the truth of the late, "different," Black, lesbian, poet, warrior, and mother Audre Lorde who said, "Your silence will not protect you." She also might have said, "Your sameness will not protect you." You are different. We are different. And that is good.

The most common responses to us as an interracial lesbian couple have been incomprehension, confusion, and confoundedness. How can you be with a woman? How can you be with a Black* woman? With a white woman? How can you consider having children? What race will they be? Sometimes, instead of the questions, there is simply silence/silencing, horror, or hope.

We are trying to have children, and again it is incomprehensible to people. There was the white doctor who whispered furtively to Mary (who is also white), "Seeing you, I just think I should tell you that this sperm specimen is Black." If it wasn't a mistake, he seemed sure that we couldn't possibly want people to know.

"You are our hope for the future," said one white colleague (also a lesbian). It seems to be a statement made with the best intentions about the impossibilities of our existence in the present. We do not want to be anyone's hope for the future, rather we want to live in the present with integrity among other different people.

"It's just too much," is one of the kinder things Mary's father's partner said when she banned Mary from ever visiting her home

---

*In resistance to whiteness as a cultural norm, Black will be spelled with a capital "B" throughout this essay.

again. Renee's family is very kind, but they just cannot think about "it;" it is too much. Thinking about race and sex at the same time is too much for them. But all over the world, lesbian, gay, bisexual, and transgendered people of color and their partners have to think about race, sex, and class every day and every night, mostly because someone else has made it an issue.

A wonderful, contemporary philosopher has made it her project to problematize that which appears normative, that which is taken for granted. Naomi Scheman asks, "How do you know that you are normal?" The answer is, "You don't; you're not; we're not!" And that is good. The problem is that whenever people define what is "normal" or typical, they usually leave some people out, either by accident or on purpose. If you are a white lesbian or gay man, what makes you think your experience is typical of all lesbian and gay people? If we are incomprehensible to people as a couple (and sometimes as individuals), that is great! It saves us from the soul-killing assumption of sameness that those who appear to be "normal" must try to live up to—their secret quirks and family skeletons always threatening to bust loose in an explosion of difference.

Not only are we different as a couple, we are different as individuals. Mary is from a white, affluent, upwardly and downwardly mobile family of divorce. Renee is from an affluent, middle-class, African-American family where blood relatives and non-blood relatives are white, Black, and many shades of brown. Both of us have other lesbian and gay relatives. Renee has lost two cousins to AIDS. At an early age, Renee knew she was different, as a Black girl attending a white, private school and as someone simultaneously excluded from and uninterested in the (mostly white) heterosexual dating scene. Mary was taught to be the same, as a white child in an integrated public school, as a person attracted to everyone. She was a cheerleader with a succession of short-term boyfriends.

Renee came out when she got to college. She had long-term relationships with women before she met Mary. Mary came out when she got to seminary. She had never had a relationship that lasted more than a few months, and her relationship with Renee was the first with a woman.

We have been together eight years. We had a commitment ceremony with family and friends almost five years ago to affirm our

differences and our togetherness. We have both felt different from
our families for a variety of reasons, but the result was usually pain
or shame. We have come to acknowledge and celebrate differences
in our own family, and the result is often joy and growth.

Our families are different in how they respond to us. Within
Mary's family, her mother has come to be an advocate. Her grandmother and extended family have been supportive of, even if not
necessarily thrilled about, our relationship. Mary's father did not
speak to her for three years after his partner "outed" Mary by
secretly taping her phone calls to Renee and then giving the tapes to
Mary's father. Renee's family has often been extremely gracious
and inclusive of Mary in family events. However, they have a hard
time with the realities. There have been significant outbursts when
Renee came out to them, and they could not bring themselves to
even reply to the invitation to our commitment ceremony. "We
might be away that weekend" was one response. They also do not
want to talk or even think about what might happen if we have
children. Renee's mother replied, "Well, I won't tell your father
that you're trying to get pregnant," despite Renee's encouragement
of her to do exactly that. Support, hostility, inclusion, and silence
are part of both families' attempts to comprehend our relationship.

In a society of few interracial relationships, which has a history
of blatant interracial sexual violence, secret loves, and the sexual
legislation of everybody (antimiscegenation laws were declared
unconstitutional by the Supreme Court only in 1967), we are definitely not "normal." We have lived in a white neighborhood where
our building superintendent thought Renee was the maid. Now we
go to a predominantly Black church where people are more interested in us as people than they are in our races or sexual preferences, although there is no illusion that race and/or sexual orientation does not matter.

St. Mary's Episcopal Church in Harlem is a congregation that is
supportive and inclusive of gay, lesbian, and bisexual people, as well
as of persons of undeclared sexual orientation. St. Mary's is definitely
not "normal," not only because of members' differences in sexual
orientation and race but also because some members are homeless,
addicts, mentally ill, or poor. Neither are these discrete categories.
Some of the mentally ill people are gay, some of the addicts are

lesbian, and the poor belong to every category. We love St. Mary's because it is a church that is different—as we are. It is a body of believers that prefers to defy the categories. As a priest and a minister, we preach about the messiness and chaos that the Gospel calls us to embrace. Understanding all people as children of God is a complicated and challenging proposition. It requires strong speech and committed action on behalf of all people, regardless of their "differentness."

We are subject to occasional homophobic comments on the street, which reminds us of the exclusion and even violence that is faced by anyone who steps outside the (hetero) sexual norms, any woman who does not have the "protection" of a man. There is also the daily insult of racism in the United States, including racism among the white lesbian, gay, bisexual, and transgendered communities. When we travel to lesbian and gay conferences or to lesbian and gay vacation spots, Renee often is one of the few people of color. We have been refused drinks, ignored entirely, and have received comments about a "dark lover." Sometimes people talk to Mary and ignore Renee, even if Renee is the one who asked the question. Some want to "hear Renee's story"; some don't. Many do not understand why we have to talk about race all the time, never linking it to their own experience as lesbian/gay/bisexual people accused of "talking about sex all the time." In our experience, white lesbian/gay/bisexual people have no more understanding or interest in race than any other white people. To avoid the topic, some respond with euphemisms such as "Sociology is so divisive," "Why can't we just talk about sexuality? That's what we have in common." But we don't—we're different, and the costs of difference are clear; the costs of sameness are hidden. The strength and joy of difference is greater than the illusory safety of sameness.

This strength in difference is what we have come to know individually and together. Being different, we have more to learn from one another, and we can complement one another's strengths and weaknesses. The political powers that promulgate enforced sameness want to annihilate difference from their own blueprint of what human life should be. However, even those forces are willing to change, to be fluid in strategy, to try different ways of convincing people to support their agenda. By encouraging and supporting the differences among those of us who are already different, we engage in a powerful strategy for survival and life. For example, in Renee's work as a chaplain for people living with HIV/AIDS, she finds a lot of people who don't fit into the usual sexual categories of "gay" or "straight." Some identify, and some don't. Many have had same-sex relationships; some have been sex workers. Renee doesn't fit into the usual categories either because she is Black. Together, we resist not only homophobic pressures, but also the racist, sexist dualisms within the self-identified gay community. Who defines what it means to be gay or lesbian? We all do! Some movement leaders see strength in sameness—sameness with one another, sameness with heterosexuals.

We do not mean to suggest that we have nothing in common with others. Mary works with Presbyterians to start discussions about racism and homophobia in churches. They are difficult discussions, but there is strength in a nascent network of people who are willing to wrestle with life's realities. It's really not "too much"; it is real life and it is good.

Because we hope for a life that is also good, we are planning to have children, both biological and adopted. Yet again this makes us different because we are lesbians and because we are interracial. Growing up as girls in this society, we were both socialized to assume that we would have children. Mary has wanted to have a baby for as long as she can remember, including when her mother was trying to raise her with non-gender-specific toys. Finally, her grandmother gave her a doll, and it was an instant favorite. Mary also tortured her mother during high school, passionately stating that she would never have an abortion if she got pregnant because she wanted to have a baby (of course she did not tell her mother that she was not having sex; her mother simply assumed it). Renee remembers a science professor in middle school who told the all-girl class that they could choose whether or not to have children. In the context of population growth as well as other important issues, he suggested that not having children was a positive and worthy choice. Thus, Renee did not think so much about having children, not until we got together, that is. We have talked a lot about it, carefully studying the choices we have.

Most people do not assume that we have thought this out. They are confused about how it could actually happen. Why do you want to have children? How will you do it? What race will they be? Don't you worry about how hard it will be for them? The response of incomprehension comes from gay and straight alike, although white people seem to be most interested in race. But, the incomprehension turns to silence and avoidance as the process has continued. We spent four years trying to conceive through artificial insemination. We experienced racism and homophobia along with the regular depersonalization of the medical profession. One doctor kept asking Renee to have her husband come in with her, despite her explicit description of our family. Another doctor told Mary that she (the doctor) didn't know if it was ethical to refer Mary for fertility tests because she was a lesbian. Our friends were silent for the most part. They were afraid to ask because they didn't know how to respond. Women who do not get pregnant are not "normal." We don't fit, so we are again incomprehensible. This difference does not put us in danger in the way that racial and sexual difference can. This difference is more isolating as we find ourselves without support from families, friends, or communities.

As we entered the adoption process, we again were confronted with the differences of sexuality and race. One large, historic New York agency claimed that no lesbians had ever come to their orientation before. As we peruse the literature, we find that African-American children are often listed as "special needs" children simply because of their race. Corruption abounds because many people stand to make money from children who are part of the child welfare systems. Foster parents and social workers have an economic stake in keeping children in the system.

We were a bit shell-shocked after our first agency orientation. Some people there were clearly interested in the economic benefits of fostering a child (you can get $1,000 per month for an infant). The social worker attempted to convince us and one other couple who had come for information about adoption to consider fostering instead. Despite our previous research, we found ourselves, perhaps naively, unaware of the bureaucratic politics at work.

After a very positive, though amusing, home visit, we were approved for adoption with one agency, and are now in an unlimited "waiting stage." Actually, only Renee was approved for adoption as a single parent. It costs a lot of money for same-sex partners to adopt as a couple. On a follow-up phone call our social worker asked, "My supervisor just wants to know what kind of partnership you have." "Domestic partners—like being married," I replied. "Oh, Ok."

The process has been difficult. Life is messy and sometimes (often?) painful. It is different from what many of us have been led to expect. But there is life, hope, and integrity in the present struggle, in living in the present every day and every night.

Anyone who has achieved a perfectly seamless identity, with no bumps or contradictions, may be no more real than an airbrushed photograph. What is real are the contradictions, within individuals and families, and the contradictions that some individuals and families pose to our neighborhoods, communities, movements, churches, synagogues, mosques, workplaces, and to our world. We are all different from the idealized norms (young, white, male, heterosexual, physically fit, and wealthy), and we all benefit from questioning and dismantling those norms. We are convinced of the truth of the late, "different," Black, lesbian, poet, warrior, and mother Audre Lorde who said, "Your silence will not protect you." She also might have said, "Your sameness will not protect you." You are different. We are different. And that is good.

We don't want to leave you with the impression that being different is only about struggle and survival. It is much more. Again, we want to have children because we love life now, not because we're hoping for an imagined future. Being an interracial lesbian family living in the present is about joy, about celebration and fun, about friendships and flexibility, about real life without the anxieties of being "found out" or being told that we're different. We already know! So, next time someone confides in you the secret of their difference—"My daughter is dating a Mexican," "My brother is dating a white guy," "My mother is a lesbian, but she's involved with a man," or "I think I might be gay or lesbian"—say, "That's wonderful, great!" Do not ignore their, or your, fears and struggles, but encourage and affirm the difference they have just confided in you. Don't just hope for the future. Live and love incomprehensibly in the present.

Be real. Be different. Be real different.

SECTION III.
RELATIONSHIPS:
TRIALS AND TRIBULATIONS

Regardless of what model of family one prefers, most folks would agree that the true test of "family" comes during times of trial or transition. Ideally, family members care enough about us to grieve when we grieve and rejoice when we rejoice. Regardless of our circumstances, they encourage us to find ourselves and to be ourselves.

Chapter 19

Spirituality and Gay Male Couples
Living in the Context of HIV/AIDS

Richard P. Hardy

In the stories of men with HIV/AIDS, we discover that within the context of the disease, gay men in relationship often find spirituality that heals. These men live life with all that it contains of pain, grief, anguish, despair, hope, joy, and wonder. They live their lives in the deepening bond of intimacy that their love provides them. They come to discover, or simply reaffirm, values that provide meaning for them. Their lives lived in these values are their spirituality, which includes their sexuality by which they incarnate their love for each other in an ecstatic way. It also includes their vision of hope and at times their despair, fear, and guilt. It includes others who are part of their family of choice. In short, their spirituality is enfleshed as any spirituality must be if it is authentic.

The gay men who love in the midst of an epidemic and have HIV/AIDS as a third party in their partnership have their spirituality affected profoundly.*

Whether one partner is infected or both partners are infected, HIV/AIDS colors how they find meaning and value. Being diagnosed as seropositive or living with AIDS, these men find their hopes and dreams shattered; there seems to be no way out of this horror. Each has his own questions about the other remaining in this relationship. One may say, "Will he leave me now?", "Will he be able to handle all the physical and emotional stress as I become more ill?" The other may ask, "How can I manage if he falls ill?"

---

*There are many men who have assisted me in this research in a variety of ways, too many to name individually. However, I would like to thank them all for their openness, integrity, and love for their fellow gay men who live with HIV/AIDS.

or "What will I do when he dies?" Throughout the process, the different stages create new hope or new despair. Day by day, each one struggles to find meaning in a context that now seems so devoid of meaning. Even if testing HIV positive is not an automatic death sentence, the question of its progression remains.

In this essay, I offer my definition of spirituality and present the values that gay male couples have discovered as they lived out their spirituality. *Spirituality is not something that we can theoretically deduce from some abstract principle or dogma and then apply exactly to any and all situations.* Rather, the only authentic way to discover and verbalize a spirituality is to implement an inductive method that looks at, listens to, and allows it to unfurl from within the experience of the people living it.

This essay is based on the experiences of gay men who are or who have been partners of persons living with HIV/AIDS.* Some of these men were HIV positive or had AIDS at the time the relationship was formed. Others were uninfected at the time. All of them remained committed to their partners until the partner's death. Some maintained a religious faith, and others were nontheists. All, however, had a spirituality that enabled them not only to go through the tragedy that had disrupted their lives, but also to be empowered to live it out in their respective situations.

Many people immediately equate spirituality with something that is "out of this world" or opposed to body or materiality. Moreover, some see it has having to do with a particular religion. For centuries, in the Western tradition anyway, ordinary people viewed spirituality as something only for monks and clergy. It had to do with prayers and rites. For some it was about self-preoccupation rather than community. Still others saw it connected with magic and sup-

---

*Although most of the subjects interviewed had no objection to having their real names used, for the sake of maintaining their privacy, their names have been changed and other identifying characteristics have been removed. At times, I may refer to published materials by partners. When I do, these references will be exactly as given by these writers. When I quote others, these are from interviews in which they agreed to participate. This chapter is extremely limited, but it is my hope to write more extensively, presenting the material that these gay men wanted to share not only with me but with others in the hope it would help them through life with HIV/AIDS.

erstition. Yet all these notions of what spirituality is and who lives a spiritual life do not approximate reality.

The words *spirituality* and *spirit* have their roots in the Latin word *spiritus,* meaning "breath" or "life principle." Contrary to common thinking, perhaps, the realm of the spiritual is not in opposition to creation or to body. Living spiritually does not mean going through life as if one is in exile in the world, while real life is heavenly and waiting for us after death. In reality, to be spiritual means to live this human life more and more deeply and more humanly. Authentic spirituality brings together a notion of full life with all that it contains of bodiliness and spirit.

Every human being desires a life that is whole and wholesome. In the process of living, persons are challenged to find that which can help them live wholly, that is to say, to find meaning in and for their lives. Sometimes the challenges come in the form of a positive event, such as success in one's career or maybe a meeting of a future life-partner. Sometimes the challenges come in the form of a negative event, such as an illness or the loss of a relationship or job. Whatever the event, questions about life, its meaning, and worth come to the fore: "What is it that I really want?" and "Can this help me to live more honestly, more authentically?"

As gay men, we face these challenges from the very beginning of our awareness of being gay. We live through a whole series of losses and positive events. Each loss forms us more and more as we respond consciously to the questions posed at any given time.[1]

Sometimes without realizing it, our lived responses put us on the path to the integration of a value that we perceive more and more clearly in life as we live it. That value moves us out of isolation and egocentricity and into a life of dynamic interrelationship.[2] Whatever positive value we perceive as that which builds us and the whole community, as gay men, we seek to make it ours. In the process, it harmonizes the various elements in our personalities so that we now see that we are not alone. Rather we are part of a community and, indeed, of a whole universe. We live our gayness in the light of this value—whatever it be—for ourselves and for all people. *But only by being authentically who we are can we find that harmony which contributes to the life of the world.* This is living spirituality.

Spirituality may be religious or nonreligious.[3] For example, a gay man may believe in God, and more specifically in Jesus Christ and his way of living, but refuse to be part of a Christian denomination. Others may choose to be part of a denomination with a specific tradition.

Others may find any religion too oppressive and disconnected from their own experience of the transcendent. Consequently, they find their value in a nontheistic (nonreligious) approach. Here the value is not a deity, but a positive, constructive, all-engulfing value. It could be compassion. It could be love. It could be creating beauty in the world. It could be concern for the world. Whatever the value, it is something that the individual pursues as a good not only for himself but also for the world.

After explaining how he had spent his life since being diagnosed with AIDS, trying to move others in AIDS activism, Michael Callen said, "First and foremost I wanted to save our lives. And I didn't believe that you could build a revolution on anything but truth—however painful and ugly that truth may be. . . . We are a noble people. It's a complete fiction that we're a people—but it's a useful fiction that I want to believe. I will die having loved my people more than I could ever, ever say."[4]

It was his determination to provide life to people that became his value. This was a key element that made him a spiritual gay man. It was this, intertwined with human love for the gay community, that was the focus of his spirituality.

In a commitment to their partners, gay men embark on a life journey with the other. Building a life together becomes a process that both partners undertake in the love they have for each other. This life is one in which each individual develops the authentic self in and through the interrelationality to which he is committed. Partners have hopes and dreams of a long life lived happily as a couple. Searching for the life that they have may have been long and difficult. It may have been a search that was desperately passionate. Yet somehow they found each other—perhaps at a time when each had given up on ever finding someone with whom he could share his life.

As their lives intertwine they, like all couples in love, discover differences that create conflict. If their life together is to survive and grow, they must face these differences and conflicts. With open and honest communication they can work them out together. The process requires a letting go of certain things to build a deeper relationship that will survive any future tragedies that life has in store for them.[7] How they face and live this process of reconciling the differences can be extremely important today in the context of HIV/AIDS. The experience of sharing a life of integrity together offers things to gay male couples that may prepare them for the violent intrusion of HIV/AIDS in their lives, but it does not make it much easier to live their love together with this intrusion.

When we enter a relationship, there is a deep spiritual communication which occurs and affects every aspect of who each one is as a partner. There develops the gradual sharing of the total being that each person is. Moreover, the intimacy expressed in opening up to the other, both spiritually and physically, requires a basic trust and hope so that what is happening becomes something substantial, affecting each person.

Now, as partner, I can no longer be an island unto myself. Rather, as partner I am living one life with the other. This new form of life creates for me an incredible hope and passion for life, which I share with my partner and which also moves out and affects the wider community. Therefore, living a spirituality within this context is living an ever-deepening human life with and for the other. It is there that I discover, moreover, the real person I am. And the other discovers the person he is—all within this relationship, which deeply affects us both. When HIV/AIDS forces itself into this relationship, the parameters change, the circumstances modify the at-oneness. However, HIV/AIDS can become a call, a challenge, to an ever-deepening, loving relationship that creates new dimensions of the spirituality of the gay male couple.* Each of us faces that call differently because each of us has a personal story.

---

*Several years ago, I wrote an article titled "The Pre-Ceremonial Couple: Reflections for a Spirituality," which appeared in *Eglise et Theologie* (January 1977). Although it concerns primarily heterosexual couples living a commitment without any official public ceremony, I also had in mind gay couples. I speak of the fact of suffering and its role in the spiritual life of the couple. There are things I would change or perhaps not say in exactly the same way today, but I think the basic ideas expressed there remain valid.

Our personal stories constitute the core of our responses to the diagnosis of HIV/AIDS of our partner and/or ourselves, and none of us can come to grips with it except in terms of who we are. And who we *are* is who we *have been*. All the previous experiences of relationships, of purely sexual acquaintances, of hopes and dreams, or relations with friends and family (both biological and of choice) help write our stories. Hence, they affect the way in which I will respond now to this new situation, which I may have suspected, perhaps feared, perhaps avoided. *Diagnosis makes us face death, and, consequently, life.*

What happens in those minutes, hours, weeks, and months after diagnosis becomes part of that story? Some of us know of the diagnosis before beginning a relationship. Some of us find out only after we have entered into partnership.

Take the story of Chris and Bud, for example. Initially, uninterested in getting into a relationship for the first time, Chris and Bud started dating after meeting in a bar. Within a few months, they decided to live together. A few years later, Bud went for an HIV test and learned that he was seropositive. After hearing of his lover's positive status, Chris expressed these feelings, "I knew he was getting his test results. I came home, and he told me. [I was] devastated in a way. I felt as devastated as I did with the death of my parents or my brother. It seemed like a death sentence. We had been in the process of house hunting, and we put that on the back burner. I got tested and tested negative. I was very much devastated by my HIV-negative result. The doctor was, I think, a little pissed off with me because I wasn't jumping for joy."

With the knowledge of the presence of HIV in their relationship, nothing could be the same again. It put a kind of block into their relationship that had to be dealt with. There is the implication that Chris thought that if he, himself, were positive, the block would be eliminated, or at least reduced. It would certainly have made things different. As difficult as that would be, nonetheless, it just might have helped him deal with things.

Being seronegative while the one you love is seropositive raises explicit questions for some about the future. For example, Lou and Edward had been in a relationship for almost seventeen years.

Edward received the results of his HIV antibody status around the twelth year of their shared life. On learning the results, Lou said,

> We went to the AIDS testing place. They would not let significant others in, and so he got his results and then came out and told me. It was like the sun had fallen out of the sky. We walked around the street for an hour or so just holding hands. I let him experience his grief, and then we walked home. In my daily life I began to think "I'm going to be alone one of these days because I'm negative." There was also a denial process—it's just that all of a sudden death was a reality. The things we had planned for the future we still talked about, but I think we both knew they wouldn't happen.

Usually partners do think about themselves and their future, especially if there is a negative HIV status. They think about trying to deal with the fact that they will be left alone without the fulfillment of the hopes and life that the two had planned to share. Their love often does not allow the healthy partner to consider the possibility of another relationship—certainly not at that point in time. Many feel that they will never have another relationship. If the partner is positive, often he feels that no one will be interested and, interestingly enough, even if the partner is negative, there is a sense that others will be too afraid of him because he was intimately involved with someone who died of AIDS complications.

However, on a relationship level, some find a certain comfort in continuing to discuss and plan for the future. In this case, it is not really denial, but a way of balancing optimism and realism. This is one of the most difficult tasks of gay male couples affected by HIV/AIDS. For Lou and Edward, facing the future enabled them to go on living and hoping, though they realized that, more than likely, their dreams could not be fulfilled. Clearly, HIV/AIDS is the constant companion of the couple.

Jack attended an AA meeting one night. As he listened to one particular speaker reveal his story, their eyes caught each other. Afterward, Sonny said to Jack, "I laid the look on you, and you didn't have a chance." After a year of dating, they decided to be partners. Jack had been in a relationship before, but Sonny had not. They embraced those differences in experience and found that their relationship slowly came together and brought them both a lot of happiness. They had moved to a new city to start a business. It was there that Sonny got tested. They were both together at work when Jack said he got a call. It was his doctor who gave him the results over the phone. It really devastated him that he was told right then and there. Jack spoke of HIV in their relationship this way: "So HIV is like a big nuisance, a big pain in the ass. Unfortunately, it's a little more serious than that, but that's how I feel. It's still there, hanging there. Almost like it's waiting—very persistent."

Although one may be constantly questioning one's own future as a partner and trying to live in the relationship almost as if nothing had happened, the threat really cannot be avoided. Like the sword of Damocles, hanging by a single hair, it dangles while the couple waits for it to drop.

Yet, even this experience, which can be fraught with darkness and despair, contains positive potential. Jack goes on to say, "Despite this awful sort of weight hanging over our heads, it's strengthened our relationship. It has made us more secure in our love for each other, which feels good."

Sharing suffering together deepens the intimacy that is at the very heart of any relationship. However, the pain, fear, and emotional upheaval remain part of this dynamic of life together. There is no denying the horror experienced. Working through that and finding and claiming one's feelings are essential. Gradually, living with HIV or AIDS becomes the key, not only for the person infected but also for the partner. How each faces it determines its positive or negative influence on the lives of them both. Some live in fear of the future, and understandably so. Some are afraid to make plans for a trip or other things because the partner might get ill at that time. But little by little, adjustments are made, and life is lived on.

"My lover was Sean," says Steve. "I knew about him before I met him. I went to a bar. I was told that he was at another bar, so I went there. I wanted to check this out. The stories I had heard about him were kind of intriguing. So, I went over to the bar, and he picked me up."

Gradually their relationship developed, and they lived together for eight years. Then came the diagnosis of HIV for Sean. Steve remembers the event:

It was kind of strange. He found out on his birthday. We had plans for the weekend, and he kept it in and didn't want to tell me right away. That Sunday, he was sitting on the couch, and I went to hold his hand, and it was really cold. I said, "Oh my God, you feel like a corpse." He just sort of laughed and then he said, "Well, I have something to tell you." He told me his last test came back positive. He went for a test because he was getting sick all the time. The part that I remember the most was when he told me I kind of backed away from him. I guess it was a natural fear or something. I thought about it after, and he started to cry, saying, "You don't have to stay if you don't want to." I just told him that as long as we were together, we'd be OK.

Spontaneous reactions that reveal fears deep within us are normal. Yet, Steve maintained his love and commitment because in Sean and in their relationship he had found something that gave him life, and he was not about to simply let it go.

After Sean's death, Steve reflected on their life together with HIV/AIDS and could say, "I still believed in love as being very powerful and that we have inner strengths that we don't know about but that only come out during some traumatic experience."

Ultimately, love is something that can break through the shock and pain and enable the couple to live through the situation. It is that love and determination, which move them to adopt or reaffirm life-giving values that become the core of their life together.

Sometimes values change, and sometimes they remain the same. But the invasive presence of HIV/AIDS forces people to look more consciously at the values on which they have based their lives. Jack illustrated this fact when he said,

We had moved to another city and dreamed about getting a business up and running and about getting rich and famous. All those things that people dream about, and we still do. I don't know if anything has changed. It's just that we realize now we're not infallible. The road may be a little more difficult, but we're still on the road to a happy destiny, and it's been "A-OK."

In response to a question concerning the values that he holds, he says,

> Honesty is one [value] we have built our relationship on. It's become very apparent to us how necessary it is. There's also an element of—I was going to say compassion but that's not it—realization (that's it) that there's a lot of diversity not only in our lives but in how we see each other and see our relationship. Allowing for that diversity to come out. We're headed down the same road but on two paths.

A sense of oneness on the journey is clear, but at the same time there is an allowance for differences. Authenticity becomes a guiding value. To be authentic implies knowing oneself and living that self in proportion to one's self-awareness. For the gay, male couple, this means realizing that there are two individuals with their personal stories and riches who come together to share one life. *This sharing is not the whittling down of both to the most common denominator.* Rather, it is the recogition and empowerment of each to be himself.

Dennis, on the other hand, came to see and experience life more intensely, indeed differently. "Probably the most important [value] was a real appreciation for life. I love the experiences of life." Dennis was an American Indian who, like his partner, was HIV positive. His background and culture had taught him about life, but facing death in both his partner and himself gave him a new insight into the marvels of life and its wonderful diversity, which he had not experienced so deeply before. Yet, this new appreciation of life and its dynamism moved him out of any sense of isolation that his situation could have easily forced upon him. Rather, his whole situation as a partner of one living with AIDS engaged him on a path of making life as beautiful as possible for his partner and others in a similar situation. This experience led him to establish a group that enabled persons living with AIDS and those affected by HIV/AIDS to find meaning in life in the face of the disease. This organization grew steadily, and it enabled others like him to find meaning.

Even today, after his own death, it thrives and offers a place for seropositive persons to find empowerment in living, not dying. Yet, his affirmation of life found expression in a more personal way as well. He became more and more a listener, and in this way he empowered others like himself to experience this life ever more profoundly. His native background and his own quiet but strong personality and his experience with his partner gave him a unique ability to relate to others in the challenges posed by HIV/AIDS. His love for life moved him outside of himself, which had important social effects both organizationally and individually.

Rick found that his partner's diagnosis affected his view of the important things in life:

> [Before the diagnosis], I guess money, getting ahead—those things were important, also traveling and enjoying life. And I think now I enjoy all those things, but they don't have the same importance. I think I'm more interested in my relationship with Phil [his partner] and friends. And I'm more interested in my relationship with people. Maybe you realize . . . maybe I'm getting older, and I'm reevaluating priorities. While these things are to be enjoyed they're not the vital issues.

Rick affirmed the good things of life. A diagnosis of HIV/AIDS does not destroy their validity and one's desire to appreciate them. However, the awareness of the presence of HIV/AIDS brought him to understand that not all things are equal in meaning. People, and his interaction with them, became much more important than the enjoyment of things. He found life primarily in a positive relationship, with his partner first of all and then with others. Seeing the life their relationship brought to him and to his partner became the primary element giving the human experience meaning. Furthermore, seeing that did not push Rick and his partner into a solipsistic outlook. Rather, because of that interrelationship, he discovered the tremendous importance and value of other human relationships. Living positively with people became something that he saw as an enhancement of his own life and relationship.

Although Rick does not mention it, other gay male couples affected by HIV/AIDS speak of deciding not to remain friends with those who created a negative, stressful situation for them. This is a very healthy move, which is usually accompanied by forming new friendships that enhance the lives of all concerned.

As we actually become conscious of the importance of other people and of having a wholistic, life-affirming relationship with them, we discover or realize more intensely that this is what living is all about. It moves us out to the world. Everything takes on a new hue and excitement. Moreover, it makes us more and more sensitive to the positive and destructive realities of living. So, we rejoice more in the life-enhancing things, especially people and the beauty of creation, and we suffer more intensely in the life-destroying experiences. The values that form the core of spirituality enable people to really *live* all that life contains.

Steve met Sean at a bar. Sean didn't believe in relationships at the time. Neither of them really expected more than a one-night stand. But within a short time, they moved in together. Only after beginning the relationship did they discover, first Sean's seropositivity, and then Steve's. Sean died of complications from AIDS eight years after their relationship began. Steve's values were different before Sean's diagnosis. Steve said, "I didn't really have any goals because I was drinking a lot. I just wanted a nice life, an easy life. I don't know . . . it was important to be financially secure, I guess, because that really worried me a lot." Then with the implications of his diagnosis things began to move him on a path of gradual change. "It made me grapple with more. Even though I didn't stop drinking at that time, I was learning a lot. All the stuff that was thrown at me. I had to try to process it all. So I learned from it." When Sean became ill, Steve found something that provided him with a key for his life: "I still believed in love as being very powerful and that we have inner strengths that we don't know about but that come out only during some traumatic experiences."

In the living out of difficult, even shocking, experiences, a person can begin a process of reflecting and become more and more aware of primary values such as love. That process opens an inner depth, and there one discovers that one has the ability to live in and through whatever it is that seems to be controlling one's life. In fact, one discovers that one can control it rather than being controlled by it.

Cyril met Louis, who had worked the streets since he was young. They developed a relationship that lasted until Louis died ten years later. The whole experience enabled them both to grow as they shared their lives together. Cyril noted,

> I try to keep faith that there's something bigger than just life on earth. This is part of life, and HIV is just another disease that came about. Of course, I feel sad at times. It makes me think that I'm not immortal and that you should live every day. Don't put off until tomorrow what you can do today and live life to the full.

He began to notice things that had always been there, but he never really saw: ". . . the colors, the wind in the trees, the snow falling. I like to go in the park and sit and look up at the stars for hours hoping to see falling stars. I talk a lot to my Higher Power, and he answers me. I feel better after I do, believe me." The whole experience of living with Louis and HIV/AIDS moved him out of his own small world into the universe.

As Louis got sicker, Cyril became preoccupied with the situation. He had to work and leave Louis home alone. He worried constantly. Louis became even more the center of his consciousness. "I was more worried about Louis than I was about myself. I was raised that way—to think of others before thinking about yourself, make other people happy. It probably got me more human."

Cyril prioritized and clarified his values. Before the diagnosis he wanted "a comfortable home, a nice relationship—a loving relationship—and to have a normal and decent life." His love for Louis deepened with each day despite the ravages of the disease. In responding to a question of his values during Louis' illness, Cyril said, "I never stopped loving him, even though his body was changing. When I met Louis, he was very muscular. I stopped looking at the physical, and I started looking inside the person. That was a big thing. If I would have met him like that there was no way I would have even touched him. But it didn't bother me to hold him, to kiss him, or to sleep with him."

The bond that had developed over their ten years together made Cyril realize that the person within remains and comes to be treasured more and more. The degeneration of Louis' body could not destroy the years of intimacy, which had prepared them both for this period. They had tapped the source of their love for each other. Yet, the pain, the suffering and the physical scarring could not be eliminated. They both had to live with it, and they did, but only because their love for each other made it possible. For Cyril, his own illness and Louis' death enabled him to say, "I don't take life for granted now. Life is a privilege. It's also a privilege to be sick because you learn things and discover things inside you that you never knew were there. And they just come, and I surprise myself." He finished by offering some advice to other surviving partners, irrespective of whether they, themselves, are living with HIV/AIDS or not, "Don't be afraid to love again."

In these stories of men with HIV/AIDS, we discover that within the context of the disease, gay men in relationship often find a spirituality that heals. These men live their lives with all that it contains of pain, grief, anguish, despair, hope, joy, and wonder. They live their lives in the deepening bond of intimacy that their love provides them. They come to discover, or simply reaffirm, values that provide meaning for them. Their lives lived in these values are their spirituality, which includes their sexuality, by which they incarnate their love for each other in an ecstatic way. It includes their vision of hope and at times their despair, fear, and guilt. It includes others who are part of their family of choice. In short, their spirituality is enfleshed as any spirituality must be if it is authentic.

Jacques Pasquier, speaking of relationships, says, "Two people are in relationship when each makes a difference to the life of the other."[6] The gay male partners to whom I have referred made a difference to the lives of the others. Those of us who have been blessed with such a relationship of significance and difference find that we express our gratitude for this gift by living it with a passion and joy, which not even HIV/AIDS can destroy.

NOTES

1. See *Coming Out Within: Stages of Spiritual Awakening for Lesbians and Gay Men—the Journey from Loss to Transformation,* by Craig O'Neill and Kathleen Ritter (HarperSanFrancisco, 1992); *Embracing the Exile: Healing Journeys of Gay Christians,* by John E. Fortunato (The Seabury Press, 1982).

2. See Sandra Schneiders, "Spirituality in the Academy," in *Modern Christian Spirituality: Methodological and Historical Essays,* by Bradley C. Hanson (Ed.) (Scholars Press, 1990, pp. 15–37).

3. See Daniel A. Helminiak, "Non-religious Lesbians and Gays Facing AIDS: A Fully Psychological Approach to Spirituality." In *Pastoral Psychology* (May 5, 1995); and "The Quest for Spiritual Values," in *Pastoral Psychology* (Winter, 1989). Also, I highly recommend the excellent book *Wrestling with the Angel: Faith and Religion in the Lives of Gay Men,* by Brian Bouldrey (Riverhead Books, 1994). Each chapter is a masterpiece of literature and reflection on religion and how some gay men relate to it.

4. Michael Callen, "The Finale," in *Genre* (February/March, 1994).

5. See *Knowing the God of Compassion: Spirituality and Persons Living with AIDS,* by Richard P. Hardy (Novalis, 1994).

6. "Healing Relationships," in *The Way* (1976, pp. 208–209).

Chapter 20

Letting Go
A View of Grief in Process
(Finding My Way Back to Me)

Jane Adams Spahr

You hurt me more than any human being I have loved and that is because I opened myself to depths of my personhood I believe I had sealed off from others. I opened myself up to loving you in a way I hadn't before. It is a strange place to be, having crafted my calendar this fall, winter, and spring, to take seriously our time together, even though you requested it a long time ago. You are now not here. My time alone clings to me and clangs deafly inside of me.

———

The candle flickers. It has been burning for seven days. I watch the flame go out and smoke waft up through the glass holder. "How do I ritualize this pain? How do I fathom she is gone?" I ask my therapist, who happens to be Jewish. A Jewish ritual after death is to burn a candle for seven days and watch the flame go out. "Janie," she said, "It will help make her leaving more real." The first candle I lit was when I helped Coni move out in August. The last time I felt this loss was over fifteen years ago when Jim, father of our children, now dear friend, and I decided to separate. I began to cry. "No," I said out loud. "No, this can't be. Not Coni and me, not Coni and Janie." This couldn't be.

Coni and I had done good therapy to be together. We were both independent and honored each other's style. We were together seven years when the call came from the Downtown Church in Rochester, New York. Our mutuality, once so easy in our work and life, living together, catapulted me out of town, traveling, moving us into a national scene. Coni at times went with me, which we both loved, but our home life, once so together, was now changed. I remember us sitting on our bathroom floor crying together. I remember her saying, "I have to do this, Janie. I have to find me." I sensed that finding her probably meant leaving me and going toward herself and possibly another.

It is different when we are going to find ourselves and are then drawn to another. This time I was being left. I didn't know this kind of pain. We had decided to take a time out, away from each other. As Coni drove away the first time, in August, I heard crying out of me that I had never heard before. It was from a place I didn't know. When she drove out of the driveway, I went to the back bedroom and cried as if the tears had been backed up all the way down to my toes.

I began a journal. I wrote four journals to Coni, from August through May.

Journal Entry, August 28, 1994:

Dear Coni, I think I may need to unpack us, to meet you again, face to face, with different knowledge. In sadness, not only does the myth explode, but idealism may take over as well. I only know the aching in my heart. I know the longing to see you, to touch you, to see your face; to be close to you again, life-partner, lover, and friend. I am to prepare two speeches today. They linger somewhere inside of me, wanting to give birth, close to the surface. Then, comes your face, you in your jogging suit, you in our bed at Diane's in the little cave, you and little Chetty dog, and I am lost in the dream of you. Tears are so close to the surface in, around, and behind my eyes. So many changes, and now emptiness. A sound deprivation without you in my heart. Heart of my heart, love of my life, I understand death, I understand dark, I understand loss, all in a whole new way, yet knowing it from so many places. Alone, strange, quiet, peaceful, knowing, I'm not bad company for myself. Still, so much noise in the silence. I need space, space to breathe, to feel, to cry, to know this new place without you. No sense, nonsense, non-sensical without you, the longing, brought up short, our breaking up affects others. Hearing others deal with their feelings, knowing our love for one another causes them to look at their relationships.

Night after night, whether on the road or at home, I lit the seven-day candle. At night I laid on my mat on the floor in our bedroom; I wanted to sleep on a mat because I wanted to be close to the ground. I wanted to be in a single, small bed, surrounded by stuffed animals. As I lay on the floor, I could see the flickering of the candle in the other room. There was something comforting about waking up in the middle of the night and seeing the light's shadows flicker. Waking up, I would lie awake from 11 p.m. to 2 or 3 a.m., processing in my mind, feeling Coni, talking with her, and talking with God.

Journal Entry, September 22, 1994:

I did not know how much I counted on being together, how much I counted on the presupposition that no matter what, we could move through whatever was dealt to us. Whatever we responded to, we could be there for and with each other. Maybe this time apart, however, is helping us deal with what has happened in a way we could not do together. You hurt me more than any human being I have loved, and that is because I opened myself to depths of my personhood I believe I had sealed off from others. I opened myself up to loving you in a way I hadn't before. It is a strange place to be, having crafted my calendar this fall, winter, and spring, to take seriously our time together, even though you requested it a long time ago. You are now not here. My time alone clings to me and clangs deafly inside of me. The lake is dark inside; I plunge into it day and night, into my being. I have never known myself so quiet or pensive. The grief overwhelms me at times. I call you when I hit the wall. It has taken me three solid days to come up for air from you staying overnight. We are so naturally, easily together. It seems so strange that you are not here. As I prepare to do a Holy Union tomorrow, I know you are somewhere else. A thud sounds in my being again. I am missing you so. I love you, Janie

THUD

Another layer deeper I am going
Falling down to another ledge
Another ledge deeper into my soul
Hello, Janie, and there you are

On the same ledge.
Each ledge deeper,
Will you be there?
Is there a place where you won't be?
Or, will I continue to the edge,
To layer deeper,
Only to see your face
Smiling back
at me.
Or, will I reach a ledge
Where only I am there,
Breathing in and out
Face to face with myself
I don't know that place yet
I only know as I crawl
Down to the next ledge
You are sitting there,
Waiting for me.
God of ledges,
Ease me down in her
Into me, into You.
The abyss waits
To fall into the abyss
Not wondering if anyone
Or anything is there.
Diving deep into the abyss,
Arms open to feel nothingness
Falling, falling
Is there a thud in the end?
Like astronauts into space
Letting go of the umbilical cord of starship
Lost in space
But finding oneself
Meeting oneself face to face
The abyss
Will you be there, too, Coni?

I had spoken often about seeing a picture in my mind's eye of us sitting around your grandparents table at the farm. You were so afraid to tell them about yourself being lesbian. Your family had made it so difficult and had asked you to swear that you would never tell your grandparents. I knew by other times when we had been with them that somehow they must have known about us by the kind of conversations we had. When your grandpa would look at me and say, "Well, who cooks the meals?" I said to you in late October that I saw a picture again. I dreamed about us sitting at your grandparents' farm table. It seemed to me the final picture I saw on the screen of our life together. We flew together. It was nice to sit together. We smiled at each other. We rented a big car so we could take them out for a ride. We could also go up to Springfield to see your mother and dad when we were there. We got the car and began to drive toward Vandalia, where we would see your cousin and aunt and uncle. You had brought some beautiful instrumentals, which we put into the car tape player. You became sleepy. I drove the car from St. Louis almost to Vandalia. I would look over and see you sleeping. The sky was crystal blue. We drove through St. Louis, then into farm country. I felt like I was seeing your life unfold before me, little farm girl, who loved to sit on the back of your grandpa's tractor. I looked at you asleep in the seat beside me and the farmlands rolled out in front of me, your herstory from a little farm girl to the present laid itself before my eyes. I looked at you and thought, "Remember this, Janie. You will never see her again like this." There was something happening inside, a way of knowing that this was our end.

Journal Entry, November, before Thanksgiving 1994:

> *Dear Coni, getting back to me*
> *To see who I really am*
> *I've been taking care of you*
> *You've been taking care of me*
> *Getting back to yourself*
> *Now get yourself back, Coni*
> *Go and find out who you are*
> *You have a family again*
> *You faced your fear*
> *You lived through it*

Your family is there for you
In ways you are just beginning to feel again
Farm girl, little girl
With a horse named Sandy
Stick horses high in the loft
Stick horses you rode through the woods
With Billy Tom
You found just the right kind of sticks
Corralled in the horses for the night
Only to begin a new day again
You were chosen to run water to Dad
An honor Mom bestowed on you
To run to the fields
To ride on the back of the tractor
To go to the sales
The horse shows
To ride with the pigs
In the open truck
To sleep with Mom and watch the stars
With your first soul-mate late at night
To hear her stories
To have your arm tickled
By Grandmother God, herself
Whiffleball player, jungle-gym climber, carousel rider
Jumping, running, throwing, catching,
Watch me do "dangerous twicks"
Little, strong, hope-filled farm girl
You gave me a memory of you
Of you and Mom and Dad
Grandparents who have significant names
Mom and Dad
Who love you with everything

We had hoped to have Thanksgiving together. That had been on our calendar. But, with us now living apart, I went to see my family. On Wednesday evening, I made Cornish hens so we could have our own Thanksgiving together. We were sad. Coni would be going off with new friends to the Russian River. I flew to Phoenix and then drove to Sun City. Chet, my youngest son, was with me. It was good to be with him. I knew he was sad that you and I were going through this hard time. That weekend with Mother and Dad, I remember lying awake from my usual time, 11 p.m. to 2 a.m., talking with you way inside. Something snapped in me one night that weekend. I began to know you were with someone new. It felt like you had met someone. I got home Sunday night and tried to reach you several times. My fear was not unfounded. I got hold of you very late, probably 2 a.m. We talked and cried together. I asked you the question; I asked you to come and talk with me, to finally say to me that I was not your partner, nor did you know if I ever would be. I asked you to come to dinner. I wanted you to tell me that our relationship as partners and lovers was no more, or I would still be hopeful. On November 29, you came to the house with our little dog, Chetty. We had dinner together, and I asked you to say those words to me. You cried with me. I said that I knew you loved me. "Of course, I always will," you said. "Then say it, Coni. Say it so I don't keep thinking we are still partners." I said to you what Jim Spahr had said to me fifteen years earlier: "I wish it were me, but it's not. And I wish it could be me, but it's not. So be free, find yourself, and find your way." I told you that I loved you with everything, and this was the hardest thing that I had ever done. To let you go, love of my life. We wept together and then you drove away.

Again, the crying was beyond anything I had ever heard inside of me, like hearing someone else sobbing. I lit another candle. That Friday I went to Chicago. I wrote this journal entry on December 2, 1994, on my way to Chicago on the plane:

> *The quiet helps when dying, when grieving*
> *It helps me listen and go inward*
> *Helps me go farther inside*
> *Farther than I've ever known*
> *I didn't know death would be peaceful*
> *My friends, most I've been with when dying*
> *Finally get to the peaceful place*
> *They've taught me about peace*
> *Missing you, Coni, is like dying*
> *Sometimes the pain is so great*
> *I wish I would die*

Other times I want night to come
So I can crawl in my bed, write in my journal,
Just let the night wrap me up in her arms
I'm not afraid at night anymore
In fact, I long for night to come
So the solitude can envelop me and hold me close
I never knew this pain of missing so badly
Missing your touch next to me like spoons
Or just being an arm's length away
But you are gone,
Gone to find yourself more
I can feel you, especially at night
I can see you in your bed
Sometimes I talk to you out loud
Other times in my mind
I wonder how you are, Coni
How school is, how therapy is going
How your life is flowing
I wonder about Mom and Dad and little Chetty dog
The holidays are coming more quickly
I have anxiety about the pain I feel
Knowing you are gone
I wonder if you miss me
I mean, I know you do and I also know
Not in the same way
Because you left awhile back
You got caught in another arena
You couldn't see me or us
You were gone
Once gone the way you were,
It's hard to come back
Still, when I saw you
When we were saying "good-bye"
You were still a fraction away
So how would I expect you
To see me or us fully?
I remember when Michael was dying
Don and I were whispering at the end of the bed
Michael put his finger to his lips, smiled, and said,

"Quiet, please."
I think he was listening to friends
Beckoning him on, to the other side
Maybe it's like watching a symphony conductor
Tap the stand, hands up
And for that moment it is all quiet
Then comes the music
I wonder if dying is that momentary pause
Then, onto the other side
I wonder how long this momentary pause will be.
How long this grieving will go on
It feels like the momentary pause
Will be a long time
When Bob was getting closer to dying
He got quieter and quieter
I asked him if it was peaceful in there
He smiled and nodded his head
I think I'll call some of our friends
From the other side
To help me and us through this time
Larry and Carol helped before
I know Bob, Marty, Michael, Steven, Nick, Gary—
The whole gang—
Understands, and they'll help
They are already helping so many of us here
Maybe it's a fine tuning to next steps of living
To die and then live again
With such a different perspective
Dying isn't so bad
What's hard now is I have to begin
To live without you
All these years of living with you
And loving you
Now, I will live without you
And that kind of dying kills me
But I'll do it, Coni,
Because I have to
Because we each have lots to do and be
I guess I'll plunge in again

But, God, I wish
Coni and I were plunging in together
Well, maybe some day
Take care of yourself, Coni
You have a lot of folks on the other side
And this side
Rooting for you and for me
And I even think, for us
I love you, Con
Janie

In December, friends and family were here. I felt like at night I didn't want to move, as though moving in bed I would crack from the inside out. After everyone went to bed, I lay awake. I needed so much space and silence. The silence was the only thing that gave me peace. My friend, Annie, came to stay while Mother and Dad were here. I laid on a mat on the floor, she on a bed across the room. "Are you awake?" I would say at 2 and again at 3 a.m. There are others, close friends, who have gone through this experience of losing a person they love, either through death or through separating. It was those friends that I needed to talk with most. I remember calling them on the phone in the day or late at night and crying with them, over and over telling the story. They knew the words before I said them, but their patience and their listening attentively helped me live. January and February were sleepless. They were times when I would wake up and feel Coni—times when I thought I would die. Thank God for friends who listened over and over again.

January 27, 2:30 p.m., on the plane coming from Rochester, New York: I'd done the first fundraiser for "That All May Freely Serve," my work in Rochester. It was a beautiful evening with snow coming down, with John Williams playing the piano. This was the first time Coni had not been with me for a fundraising event such as this. I always introduced her as my partner and friend. This is the journal entry I wrote:

FEELING SINGULAR

Dear Coni,
Not to be calling you each night I am gone
Not to hear your voice and share

What we each are doing
Wondering how you are, how Chetty is
Wondering what your life is like
Coming home again on the plane
Feeling anxious and alone
Walking into the house, lying on the mat, looking at the wolves
Where to find solace in my soul
Only the One who dreamed us into being
Remember when you would say that
She and the wolves looking back at me
Reaching inside of me, only they are safe
You are no longer safe
You who I let hold me
You, who said you would always be there
The knowing inside, did I know
The first fundraiser
With "That All May Freely Serve"
Music from Gay Men's Chorus Quartet
Their words, "And there you were in my mind"
All those years, all those fundraisers
And there you were
Then reeling inside, smiling to you, a nod
But, you weren't there this time
Feeling singular, walking to the podium, feeling singular
From Coni into community, stepping into the microphone
                alone
I never fathomed my life without you
You, my soul-mate, lover, friend
You are gone
How come you still live in me
I can't get over you
I can only go through you
Through the eye of the storm
I'm in the middle of it
I want to get to the other side
My grief holds me, spinning me, finally, into me
Is that what happens, Coni?
Is that what time does?
Will it bring me peace?

The peace I see when I pray with John or Hilton
Will it be a way of knowing
Oh, I know the "we-ness" of us, of you, sweet, beautiful Coni
The "I-ness" is so different, so mysterious
Gliding through a labyrinth deep inside of me
Letting it all go, listening
Not even being able to respond
Listening to the flames in the wood fire
Listening into the eyes of a large she wolf
Listening to silence on my mat
The longing for no sound
Safe is in me, soundless me
The one who travels from the mat
Can you hear me, Coni?
There is no sound
Can you hear me?
I still see you
I still hear you in the no-sound place
Stillness, a longing for stillness in my soul
I walked to the podium and I felt singular

Journal Entry, February 13, 1995:

Dear Coni, I look from a different perspective now, as I float into Valentine's Day, skittish, worried a little, trying to protect a little, putting my arm up from the inside, waiting to be hit with a feeling I don't want. A strange feeling from the inside, like turning a radio dial, the seek button, afraid, skittish about what feeling I'll tune into. That is my work, the map inside to be explored. It's expansive inside here. I need lots of room to breathe, lots of room to stretch. Grief does that. It's like God, please give me room, inside and outside. I don't like clutter either. Clutter gets in the way of wanting to embrace vastness. Vastness helps me hold the particularity, the particular feeling that hurts. The gradation of each part of hurt. The healing is done by gradations, level into level into level. I pray, "Space, open me into your extraordinary vastness so I can rest and hold the graded feelings and not lose my mind or lose my heart." Out there, in the universe and in here, Coni, we connected. That is why unhooking is so difficult for me. The connection was more than us. Out there, in here, I still feel you. I still see your face. I feel the pulse of you. Is that my twining gone awry? But why does it feel like a former kind of knowledge out there in here? Somehow, I believe if I walked out into space, I'd see you there smiling to me. Then, we could begin again on another level.

I had begun to collect pictures of wolves, and people began sending me cards with wolves on them, wolves in the snow. Looking at these pictures of the wolves seemed to be my only solace. I put these pictures up in front of my desk on the wall. I look at them every day.

Journal Entry, early March 1995:

My journey is with wolves in the snow
Who have visited me twice at night
Once on the mat and once by the backroom bed
And still the she wolf and the She God
Know how to soothe my soul
When everything and everyone seems to be
In another reality
It is a place I've never been before
A fragile place for me, but not a scary one
A place unto its own
Where humans seem far away
A place where wolves and God roam
A place where they are on the alert
For those who cry out in the night
I never knew this place existed
Maybe that's where you go when
You have been so down, Coni
I wonder if you have been there
Or, if you let yourself know the lake
Your beautiful black lake inside
I think introverts must smile
At us extroverts
You have probably been swimming in the dark lake
A long time
There is so much to share together
How I want to share these trips, these times

With you
How much I want to hear of you
Your growth and your life
And then the pain
The knowing you are not where I am
You are working on your stuff with another now
And I am on a different journey
Oh, Coni, I love people, probably deeper
I just miss one
I miss you, Coni
I think you feared touching other souls
You thought it should be only one
There are many people we touch along the way
I chose to go in and on the way with you
Take care of you, Coni, and Chetty
I saw Chetty in a dream last night
He looked like a perky, shiny, gray and white pup
His fur was glowing
I hope you and he are talking together at night
He loves you so
I hope you are learning and growing
I'll see you in the stars
I'm loving you,
Can you ever know how much I miss you?
You do your work,
Learn, and be free.
I am doing my work to individuate.
Each day, individuating,
Unlocking from starship, astral planing to you from the stars.
Janie

In March, I had just returned from Rochester. I was returning the phone calls in the early morning when my call waiting rang, and I heard a voice and someone crying. I knew the voice immediately. It was Coni. Something in her voice made me shake. She said that our little dog, Chetty was very sick, that he was dying, and that she might have to put him to sleep. Would I come and be with her and with him? I went to the vet's in the early afternoon. Chetty was in a cage on the floor. They opened the cage, and I was able to lie down on the floor and hold him. He crawled right up to me. Little boy was so sick. I talked to him for a long time. He lay there. I was there about an hour, and Coni came in. She kneeled down and touched him and touched me. The doctor came in and talked to us about Chetty. We loved him and held him. She knew that she had to put him to sleep. We took him together into the doctor's office and loved him and held him and thanked him for his wonderful life, and then we put him to sleep. We carried him to the car, brought him into the house. We wanted him to be buried here. We dug a hole in the backyard, and then we held him and loved him. We said a prayer, thanked him and God, and buried him in the ground. We came back into the house very quietly. "I love you, Janie," she said. We walked out the door, and there was her little maroon Mazda. I said, "You know, Chetty and I had a lot in common. We loved you unconditionally." I could see the pain and love in her eyes. She told me she loved me, and I told her I loved her. In many ways, she can't believe we're not together, either. She drove away again. I came back into the house. I went to the backyard, and I sat there with Chetty. There are still days when I take moments and sit out there with him.

Sometimes at night I sleep in the back room. Actually, I sleep all over the house. When I am restless, I don't know where to lay my head. But there is something comforting about sleeping in the back room, knowing that Chetty's grave is not far away. Burying Chetty in our backyard was very symbolic for me.

From August 1994 to May 1995, I faithfully wrote journals to Coni. The four journals are now on my shelf, and I have left instructions that if anything were ever to happen to me that Coni should get them. In late May, I knew it was time for me to begin to write my own thoughts, my own dreams, my own life, to separate farther from Coni. It was strange to begin writing in a journal that was only for me. I felt disloyal.

Journal Entry, May 10, 1995:

Dear Coni, I have to come out again. I have to come out and say and live again without you, even in the recesses of my being. I have to come out alone and be alone. I have to know what that feels like. I have to say who I am and where I am. I have to grow into Janie again. I have to go back before you, into you, and through you into me again.

My therapy: by the time I came back from New York City in June, where we had been together a year earlier at the Gay Games, and I had stayed at the convent again, something was happening in me. The grief had plummeted me so far that all I could feel was pain. Rising out of the ashes, I of course had to begin looking at me, to begin unpacking my family systems; to begin looking at why I choose, who I choose, and why I do what I do. I began to separate more clearly what was Coni's emotionalwork and what was mine. I wanted to know what it was to individuate, having been a twin, and then partnered with people all through my life. I began to read the *Tibetan Book of the Dead.* I looked inside and realized I was learning how to live again, but it was learning how to die as well. My friends who have crossed to the other side have been my greatest teachers. I think I have in some way known death with Coni's leaving. I must learn to die before I can live. For a twin, it is to separate from that kind of communion that I longed for with another.

It was in June, in the convent, that I wrote the following journal entry:

Relationships take on different meaning now for me, as I begin again to breathe. The intricacies of relationships seem burdensome. The exhaustion has set in from a year highlighted everywhere by the loss of you. I feel like those little animals who live underground, who pop up in different places saying, "I'm here. No, I'm over here. No, over here." Coming from deep places underground, emerging when there seems safety.

Yet, life is not safe. Risks help us grow. When the earth moves, foundations shake, and our relationship was foundational for me. It was a trusting of reality, a framework I came to know as true. In a real way now, you have died, and we have died. The foundation has shaken, yet now you are living, and so am I. They call this transition "grief work."

The weekend of my fifty-third birthday, I was at the Christian Lesbians Out Together Conference (CLOUT). I got more in touch with my part of Coni's and my relationship and what I needed to work on about not recreating my family system, about learning this individuating that seems almost impossible.

Journal Entry, August 12, 1995:

Dear Coni, Today one year ago, we sat at the beach at Point Reyes. I said good-bye to you and invited you to move on and do what you felt you had to do. Was that what was expected? We said we would not hold on, so another piece, another layer falls open. You are not here at CLOUT, but you are. I miss you, Coni. I miss our friendship, the holding at night, your car coming in the driveway, the nod across the room. Today, I am fifty-three years old. Why is it I feel you, still listen for you in my heart. Still wonder where and how you are. I love you, Coni, I always will. Now let go of me, Coni. Find your voice. I am becoming very different, a different Janie.

I spoke with Coni in early September about coming to get the rest of her things out of the house. In a way, it was an illusion to have her things there. In a way, it made me think there was the possibility of some hope, even though I knew she wasn't coming back. She understood. She said she would have the things gone by the end of September. She would take them while I was away. On Friday, September 29, when I was in Rochester, Coni Staff took all her belongings out of our home. A portion of her note, which was on my desk, said, "Dearest Janie, Again, hard. The final movement of 'things,' and it means so much more . . . hard, very hard. I am glad you are back with friends in Rochester who love you so much. You have so, so many places, people who care for you and cared for you and me. I love you very, very much and I was so glad to talk with you on the phone Wednesday night. Thank you. The ultimate part doesn't change. It's true, simply true. Talking to you as we both grow, *Coni*."

In a corner of the letter it says, "Leaving the key is probably the hardest. I love you."

Journal Entry, October 6, 1995:

Dear Coni, Your letter sits on my desk. Expectantly, I read it, trying to read what is way underneath and while all the material things are gone. Now, I will reclaim my house, which once was filled with you and me. Day and nights, nights and days of us. Our house. The house moves from us back to me. How to ritualize you away from memories of you everywhere. You say you are making your way back to you. You say you leaned heavily on me. Find you, Coni Staff. Find who you are. I, too, am finding my way back to me. I don't want to go through this kind of pain ever again. I'm on a journey way inside here. Reaching out tonight would not do it. Reaching in, letting the night come to me in the quiet where I can listen and hear God to the silence, which has so much noise. I guess you knew that. There are days and nights filled with friends who really care, friends and family. Oh, God of the wolves, come tonight and lie next to me. You have a way, when night is here, to still me. I trust you and the she wolf. The she wolf and the She God seem to know when to come visit. What a time this is, never to be there again. Goodnight, Coni. Good-bye, dearest in my heart. You and I cannot meet now. We are on different roads. "May the She God and the she wolf bless you with yourself" (Dostoevski).

October 9, 1995, a final candle flickers in the den, and on my mat I watch the shadows. One more time I light a seven-day candle and when it is finished, I will take the burned candle, as I have done with so many, out to my barbecue pit and smash it against the brick. Then I will pick it up and throw it away. It is a long road back to me. I am inching my way back. My chest is going up and down, and I am breathing again. One more time this Jewish ritual. I will see the smoke wind its way up through the glass, and I will believe one more time, one more level, that Coni Staff is no longer with Janie Spahr. One more level down into me.*

---

*On Halloween 1995, Coni and I spoke on the phone about this essay and said that one day when the healing moves us farther along, we will write another essay together about our journey of love, friendship, loss, and deep connection.

Index

AIDS/HIV, 17-18,24-26,29,69,74,
    97,104,124,130-132,148,
    161,193,207,210,244,
    253-266
Altman, Dennis, 4
Ānanda, 122
Aquinas, Thomas, 198
Aristotle, 176
Auden, W.H., 31
Augustine, 11,67,197

Ba'al Shem Tov, 135
Baehr v. Lenin, 90. *See also* Marriage,
    Hawaii Supreme Court
Bailey, D.S., 25
Ballard, Paul, 170
Biale, David, 174
Blake, William, 123
Body Electric School, 236
Book of Common Prayer, 86
Book of Ruth, 51-60
    Boaz, 39,54-59
    Naomi, 53-59,131,173,175
    Ruth, 39,52-59,131,173-175
Boswell, John, 26,103
Bowers v. Hardwick, 7
Boys in the Band, The, 116
Breast cancer, 98,104
Brown, Murphy, 3
Browning, Frank, 202,207
Brownsworth, Victoria, 92
Buddhism, 73
    American, 125-126
    Buddhist marriage ceremony,
        118-119,124-125
    Sakyamuni the Buddha, 115,119
    Soko Gakkai, 124-125

Buddhism *(continued)*
    Wangyal, Geshe Nagwang,
        116-118
    Zen, 72,116,126

Callahan, Sidney, 200
Callen, Michael, 256
Campbell, Douglas A., 146
Chavurah, 132
Christianity, 8-11,21-23. *See also*
        Jesus
    Catholic, 6,15,31,43-44,61-75,
        97,148,163,195,218
    Christian Lesbians Out Together
        Conference (CLOUT), 284
    Christian right, 3,6,11,16,19,229,
        233,237-238
    and sexual ethics, 197-214
    Episcopal, 79-94,177,233,245
    eunuchs, 44-46
    MCC. *See* Metropolitan
        Community Church
    Quaker, 98
Chrysostom, John, 198
Clark, J. Michael, 207-208
Clinton, Hillary Rodham, *xviii*
Clinton, William Jefferson, *xviii*
Coming out, 4,53,135
Concubine, 32,39-40
Countryman, L. William, 138

Dalai Lama, 125
Dass, Ram, 73-74
David and Jonathan, 173
Davidoff, Robert, 90
Dead Man Walking, 29
Dole, Bob, 84

287

Order Your Own Copy of
This Important Book for Your Personal Library!

OUR FAMILIES, OUR VALUES
Snapshots of Queer Kinship

_____ in hardbound at $49.95 (ISBN: 0-7890-0234-5)

_____ in softbound at $19.95 (ISBN: 1-56023-910-7)

COST OF BOOKS_____

OUTSIDE USA/CANADA/
MEXICO: ADD 20%_____

POSTAGE & HANDLING_____
(US: $3.00 for first book & $1.25
for each additional book)
Outside US: $4.75 for first book
& $1.75 for each additional book)

SUBTOTAL_____

IN CANADA: ADD 7% GST_____

STATE TAX_____
(NY, OH & MN residents, please
add appropriate local sales tax)

FINAL TOTAL_____
(If paying in Canadian funds,
convert using the current
exchange rate. UNESCO
coupons welcome.)

☐ **BILL ME LATER:** ($5 service charge will be added)
(Bill-me option is good on US/Canada/Mexico orders only;
not good to jobbers, wholesalers, or subscription agencies.)

☐ Check here if billing address is different from
shipping address and attach purchase order and
billing address information.

Signature_____

☐ **PAYMENT ENCLOSED: $**_____

☐ **PLEASE CHARGE TO MY CREDIT CARD.**

☐ Visa   ☐ MasterCard   ☐ AmEx   ☐ Discover
☐ Diner's Club

Account # _____

Exp. Date _____

Signature _____

Prices in US dollars and subject to change without notice.

NAME _____

INSTITUTION _____

ADDRESS _____

CITY _____

STATE/ZIP _____

COUNTRY _____ COUNTY (NY residents only) _____

TEL _____ FAX _____

E-MAIL_____
May we use your e-mail address for confirmations and other types of information? ☐ Yes   ☐ No

Order From Your Local Bookstore or Directly From
The Haworth Press, Inc.
10 Alice Street, Binghamton, New York 13904-1580 • USA
TELEPHONE: 1-800-HAWORTH (1-800-429-6784) / Outside US/Canada: (607) 722-5857
FAX: 1-800-895-0582 / Outside US/Canada: (607) 772-6362
E-mail: getinfo@haworth.com
PLEASE PHOTOCOPY THIS FORM FOR YOUR PERSONAL USE.

BOF96

OVERSEAS DISTRIBUTORS OF HAWORTH PUBLICATIONS

AUSTRALIA
Edumedia
Level 1, 575 Pacific Highway
St. Leonards, Australia 2065
(mail only) PO Box 1201
Crows Nest, Australia 2065
Tel: (61) 2 9901–4217 / Fax: (61) 2 9906-8465

CANADA
Haworth/Canada
450 Tapscott Road, Unit 1
Scarborough, Ontario M1B 5W1
Canada
(Mail correspondence and orders only. No returns or telephone inquiries. Canadian currency accepted.)

DENMARK, FINLAND, ICELAND, NORWAY & SWEDEN
Knud Pilegaard
Knud Pilegaard Marketing
Mindevej 45
DK-2860 Soborg, Denmark
Tel: (45) 396 92100

ENGLAND & UNITED KINGDOM
Alan Goodworth
Roundhouse Publishing Group
62 Victoria Road
Oxford OX2 7QD, U.K.
Tel: 44–1865–521682 / Fax: 44–1865-559594
E-mail: 100637.3571@CompuServe.com

GERMANY, AUSTRIA & SWITZERLAND
Bernd Feldmann
Heinrich Roller Strasse 21
D–10405 Berlin, Germany
Tel: (49) 304–434–1621 / Fax: (49) 304–434–1623
E-mail: BFeldmann@t-online.de

JAPAN
Mrs. Masako Kitamura
MK International, Ltd.
1–50–7–203 Itabashi
Itabashi–ku
Tokyo 173, Japan

KOREA
Se–Yung Jun
Information & Culture Korea
Suite 1016, Life Combi Bldg.
61–4 Yoido–dong
Seoul, 150–010, Korea

MEXICO, CENTRAL AMERICA & THE CARIBBEAN
Mr. L.D. Clepper, Jr.
PMRA: Publishers Marketing & Research Association
P.O. Box 720489
Jackson Heights, NY 11372 USA
Tel/Fax: (718) 803–3465
E-mail: clepper@usa.pipeline.com

NEW ZEALAND
Brick Row Publishing Company, Ltd.
Attn: Ozwald Kraus
P.O. Box 100–057
Auckland 10, New Zealand
Tel/Fax: (64) 09–410–6993

PAKISTAN
Tahir M. Lodhi
Al-Rehman Bldg., 2nd Fl.
P.O. Box 2458
65–The Mall
Lahore 54000, Pakistan
Tel/Fax: (92) 42–724–5007

PEOPLE'S REPUBLIC OF CHINA & HONG KONG
Mr. Thomas V. Cassidy
Cassidy and Associates
470 West 24th Street
New York, NY 10011 USA
Tel: (212) 727–8943 / Fax: (212) 727–8539

PHILIPPINES, GUAM & PACIFIC TRUST TERRITORIES
I.J. Sagun Enterprises, Inc.
Tony P. Sagun
2 Topaz Rd. Greenheights Village
Ortigas Ave. Extension Tatay, Rizal
Republic of the Philippines
P.O. Box 4322 (Mailing Address)
CPO Manila 1099
Tel/Fax: (63) 2–658–8466

SOUTH AMERICA
Mr. Julio Emõd
PMRA: Publishers Marketing & Research Assoc.
Rua Joauim Tavora 629
São Paulo, SP 04015001 Brazil
Tel: (55) 11 571–1122 / Fax: (55) 11 575-6876

SOUTHEAST ASIA & THE SOUTH PACIFIC, SOUTH ASIA, AFRICA & THE MIDDLE EAST
The Haworth Press, Inc.
Margaret Tatich, Sales Manager
10 Alice Street
Binghamton, NY 13904–1580 USA
Tel: (607) 722–5857 ext. 321 / Fax: (607) 722–3487
E-mail: getinfo@haworth.com

RUSSIA & EASTERN EUROPE
International Publishing Associates
Michael Gladishev
International Publishing Associates
c/o Mazhdunarodnaya Kniga
Bolshaya Yakimanka 39
Moscow 117049 Russia
Fax: (095) 251–3338
E-mail: russbook@online. ru

LATVIA, LITHUANIA & ESTONIA
Andrea Hedgecock
c/o Iki Tareikalavimo
Kaunas 2042
Lithuania
Tel/Fax: (370) 777-0241 / E-mail: andrea@soften.ktu.lt

SINGAPORE, TAIWAN, INDONESIA, THAILAND & MALAYSIA
Steven Goh
APAC Publishers
35 Tannery Rd.
#10–06, Tannery Block
Singapore, 1334
Tel: (65) 747–8662 / Fax: (65) 747–8916
E-mail: sgohapac@signet.com.sg

7/97